Mastering Oral & Maxillofacial Surgery

Final membership exams can be a significant challenge for trainees, particularly with the increasing prevalence of single best answer (SBA) components. Many candidates struggle with this format due to a lack of targeted resources aligned with the oral and maxillofacial surgery syllabus. This essential revision tool bridges that gap, providing expertly curated SBA practice questions designed to enhance understanding and refine exam technique.

Covering key topics across oral and maxillofacial surgery, it also provides valuable insights for professionals in related specialties, including dentistry, plastic surgery, ENT, and emergency medicine.

Mastering Oral & Maxillofacial Surgery includes dedicated sections on head and neck surgery, facial aesthetics, cleft lip and palate, and advanced oral surgery techniques. This resource is tailored to both trainees and experienced surgeons looking to expand their expertise.

Mastering
Oral & Maxillofacial Surgery
A Comprehensive SBA Exam Guide

Abdul Ahmed and Ian Jenkyn

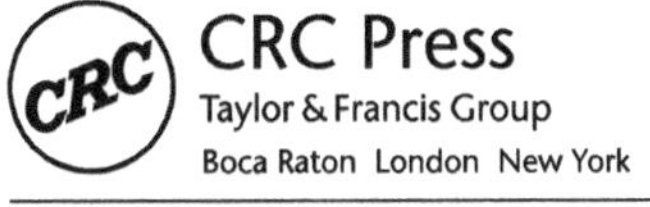

CRC Press is an imprint of the
Taylor & Francis Group, an **informa** business

Designed cover image: Shutterstock

First edition published 2026
by CRC Press
2385 NW Executive Center Drive, Suite 320, Boca Raton FL 33431

and by CRC Press
4 Park Square, Milton Park, Abingdon, Oxon, OX14 4RN

CRC Press is an imprint of Taylor & Francis Group, LLC

ISBN: 978-1-041-00320-5 (hbk)
ISBN: 978-1-041-01292-4 (pbk)
ISBN: 978-1-003-60930-8 (ebk)

DOI: 10.1201/9781003609308

Typeset in Times
by SPi Technologies India Pvt Ltd (Straive)

To my beloved wife, Shabana,
Your love, patience, and unwavering support have been the foundation of this journey. Your encouragement on even the toughest days kept me going, and I am endlessly grateful for your belief in me. This book would not have been possible without you by my side.

To my wonderful children, Maryam and Raheem,
You are my greatest inspiration. Your curiosity, laughter, and boundless energy remind me every day why I do what I do. I hope this book shows you that with dedication and passion, anything is possible.
Abdul Ahmed

To Naomi, Claire, Helen and Roger, without whose support this remarkable journey would never have been possible.
Ian Jenkyn

Contents

Acknowledgements

We would like to express our sincere gratitude to Chantal Burgess, Mohammed Bajalan, Keval Shah, Kohmal Solanki, Zahra Al-Asaadi, and Omar Sheikh for their invaluable assistance in reviewing the questions and answers throughout this textbook. We truly appreciate their time and effort in making this resource as reliable and effective as possible.

About the Authors

Professor Abdul Ahmed is a Consultant in Oral and Maxillofacial Surgery and Head & Neck Surgery at London Northwest Healthcare University NHS Trust and Chelsea and Westminster NHS Foundation Trust. With over a decade of experience as a consultant in OMFS and Head & Neck Surgery, he adopts an innovative approach to his practice, integrating cutting-edge technologies such as 3D planning, augmented reality, and robotic surgery.

A prolific author, Prof Ahmed has written multiple textbooks on maxillofacial surgery, microvascular surgery, and head and neck cancer. His commitment to education extends to teaching engagements at various universities, where he leads courses in microvascular surgery, reconstructive surgery, and undergraduate/postgraduate training. Additionally, he is a national and international speaker, delivering lectures and conducting specialised courses worldwide.

Prof Ahmed also plays a key role in surgical education and governance. He serves as the Regional Specialty Advisor for the Royal College of Surgeons and as an Educational Supervisor for the London School of Surgery.

Ian Jenkyn is currently an Oral and Maxillofacial Surgery trainee. He studied dentistry at the University of Bristol, graduating with distinction, academic awards, and the faculty's Gold Medal. He then studied graduate medicine at the University of Cambridge, graduating with distinction and academic awards. He has held several roles in medical education, most notably as a teaching supervisor of undergraduate medicine at the University of Cambridge.

Introduction

Success in exams often hinges on not just how much you know, but how effectively you apply that knowledge under pressure. This book has been meticulously designed to help oral and maxillofacial surgeons navigate the challenging world of single best answer (SBA) questions with confidence. While rooted in the UK OMFS curriculum with similar style questions to the FRCS Part A examination, this resource is not a simple mock paper but a learning tool to strengthen your foundational knowledge, refine your exam technique, and deepen your understanding of the specialty.

One of the key aims of this book is to help you identify areas of weakness or knowledge gaps that may have previously gone unnoticed. Through a diverse selection of high-yield SBA questions, we provide a structured approach to consolidating your understanding of OMFS. The breadth of content spans core areas of the specialty. It is loosely mapped to the UK curriculum and is designed to help trainees at all stages.

Time pressure is one of the greatest challenges when facing SBAs in an exam setting. This book not only develops your knowledge base but also equips you with strategies for efficiently analysing and answering questions under strict time constraints. By engaging with the questions and explanations provided, you will practice key skills such as eliminating distractors, recognising patterns in clinical presentations, and interpreting the most likely correct answer.

While primarily intended for OMFS trainees preparing for high-stakes exams, the overlapping content is also of benefit to oral surgery, ENT, and plastic surgery trainees who share common anatomical, diagnostic, and procedural areas of practice.

Where applicable, references to key textbooks, guidelines, and journal articles are included, signposting additional resources and encouraging you to engage with high-quality materials as part of your broader revision strategy.

Above all, this book is designed to be a practical, supportive tool for trainees. Whether you are in the early years of specialty training and building a strong foundation, or in the later stages preparing for the FRCS Part A exam, this resource will help you consolidate your knowledge, refine your exam technique, and approach SBAs with clarity and confidence. While exams may be a milestone, they are not the ultimate goal. This book aims to enhance your understanding and skills, helping you grow into a well-rounded clinician ready to meet the demands of modern oral and maxillofacial surgery.

DOI: 10.1201/9781003609308-1

1 Head and Neck Oncology

QUESTIONS

Q1. A 56-year-old male with a 20 pack-year smoking history and normal alcohol intake presents with a mixed red and white lesion on the left buccal mucosa. A biopsy is performed, and the histopathology report confirms epithelial dysplasia. Which of the following findings is consistent with epithelial dysplasia according to the World Health Organization (WHO) criteria?

A. Uniform epithelial stratification with orderly nuclear arrangement
B. Loss of polarity of basal cells
C. Absence of mitotic figures in all epithelial layers
D. Uniform nuclear size and shape (no pleomorphism)
E. Increased cellular cohesion with no keratinisation

Q2. A 63-year-old male with a long history of smoking presents with a non-healing ulcer on the floor of the mouth. Biopsy confirms poorly differentiated squamous cell carcinoma. CT reveals invasion of the mandible and cervical lymphadenopathy. Which feature most strongly predicts the need for adjuvant radiotherapy?

A. Tumour size >4 cm
B. Mandibular invasion
C. Nodal metastasis with extranodal extension
D. Poor differentiation
E. Invasion of floor of the mouth

Q3. An 83-year-old male presents with a painless neck lump in the level III region. Fine-needle aspiration reveals brown fluid. What is the most likely diagnosis?

A. Thyroglossal duct cyst
B. Branchial cleft cyst
C. Cystic metastasis from papillary thyroid carcinoma
D. Cystic degeneration of a lymph node metastasis
E. Parathyroid adenoma

Q4. A 62-year-old male with a 40-pack-year smoking history presents with a mass at the base of his tongue. Human papillomavirus (HPV) status is determined to be positive. How does this influence the prognosis?

A. Worsens prognosis due to aggressive tumour biology
B. Improves prognosis due to better response to treatment
C. Has no impact on prognosis
D. Worsens prognosis due to increased metastatic spread
E. Requires immediate palliative care

DOI: 10.1201/9781003609308-2

Q5. A 55-year-old male with locally advanced head and neck squamous cell carcinoma (HNSCC) is undergoing concurrent chemoradiation. The oncologist discusses potential chemotherapy agents, including cisplatin, cetuximab, and 5-fluorouracil (5-FU). Which of the following statements about these chemotherapy drugs is true?
A. Cisplatin inhibits thymidylate synthase to block RNA synthesis.
B. Cetuximab acts by targeting the extracellular domain of EGFR and may cause acneiform skin rash.
C. 5-Fluorouracil (5-FU) is a monoclonal antibody with immune-mediated cytotoxic effects.
D. Cisplatin's toxicity profile includes only ototoxicity and nephrotoxicity.
E. Cetuximab has been shown to provide superior efficacy compared to cisplatin in all settings of HNSCC treatment.

Q6. A 50-year-old woman presents with a solitary thyroid nodule. Fine-needle aspiration biopsy reveals cells with nuclear grooves and "Orphan Annie eye" nuclei. What is the most likely diagnosis?
A. Papillary thyroid carcinoma
B. Follicular thyroid carcinoma
C. Medullary thyroid carcinoma
D. Anaplastic thyroid carcinoma
E. Thyroid adenoma

Q7. A 34-year-old female presents with a 2 cm thyroid nodule. Ultrasound shows a hypoechoic lesion with microcalcifications. Fine-needle aspiration cytology (FNAC) results reveal malignant cells and small- to medium-sized follicles with colloid. What is the next best step in management?
A. Observation with follow-up ultrasound
B. Total thyroidectomy
C. Referral to palliative care
D. Radioactive iodine therapy
E. Core needle biopsy

Q8. A 58-year-old male presents with a destructive lesion involving the body of the mandible and a history of oral squamous cell carcinoma. Imaging shows cortical bone destruction. What is the most appropriate surgical management?
A. Marginal mandibulectomy
B. Rim resection
C. Segmental mandibulectomy
D. Radical mandibulectomy
E. Curettage

Q9. A 55-year-old patient with biopsy-proven melanoma of the hard palate presents with no clinical signs of regional lymph node involvement. The tumour is staged as clinically N0. The patient is otherwise healthy and has no other significant risk factors. Which of the following is the most appropriate next step in management?
A. Observation without further intervention
B. Elective neck dissection
C. Sentinel lymph node biopsy (SLNB)
D. Postoperative adjuvant radiotherapy
E. Immediate full-thickness skin grafting

Q10. A 62-year-old patient presents with a large, firm mass in the left level II cervical lymph node. No primary tumour has been found on clinical examination. The patient undergoes fine-needle aspiration of the lymph node, which confirms the presence of squamous cell carcinoma (SCC). The patient is diagnosed with squamous cell carcinoma of unknown primary (SCCUP).
Which of the following is the most appropriate surgical approach to investigate potential primary sites?
A. Bilateral palatine tonsillectomy
B. Ipsilateral palatine tonsillectomy with or without lingual tonsillectomy
C. Random biopsy of the oral cavity and nasopharynx
D. Intraoperative advanced visualisation of the mucosal surfaces with random biopsy of the larynx
E. Bilateral lingual tonsillectomy

Q11. A 49-year-old patient with SCCUP and unilateral cervical lymphadenopathy has undergone diagnostic imaging and biopsies, which show involvement of level II nodes. No primary tumour has been identified. A multidisciplinary team discusses the appropriate treatment plan. Which of the following is true for the management of the neck?
A. No surgery; proceed with radiotherapy alone
B. Neck dissection of levels IIA, III, and IV
C. Total laryngectomy with neck dissection
D. Routine dissection of all cervical nodal levels
E. Unilateral neck dissection and adjuvant radiotherapy

Q12. A 58-year-old male with a 30-pack-year smoking history presents with a leucoplakia on the lateral border of his tongue. Biopsy confirms severe dysplasia. He has poorly controlled type 2 diabetes and chronic obstructive pulmonary disease. What is the most appropriate management strategy for this patient?
A. Observation with regular follow-up every six months
B. Surgical excision of the lesion
C. Topical steroid treatment
D. CO_2 laser ablation
E. Immediate radiotherapy to the lesion site

Q13. A 60-year-old patient with SCCUP presents with bilateral cervical lymphadenopathy. The patient's biopsies confirm SCC, and the clinical team is considering the next step in treatment. The patient has not been found to have a primary tumour after extensive evaluation. Which of the following is the most appropriate treatment approach for this patient?
A. Radiotherapy targeting the bilateral neck nodes and mucosal regions at risk
B. Chemotherapy with cisplatin and radiotherapy to the neck
C. Neoadjuvant chemotherapy followed by surgery
D. Observation with regular follow-up and no immediate treatment
E. Radiotherapy targeting only the gross disease in the neck

Q14. A 49-year-old patient with SCCUP and unilateral cervical lymphadenopathy has undergone diagnostic imaging and biopsies, which show involvement of level II nodes. No primary tumour has been identified. A multidisciplinary team discusses the appropriate treatment plan. Which of the following is true for the management of the neck?

A. Radiotherapy is always preferred over surgery for unilateral, small-volume neck disease.
B. Bilateral neck disease without extranodal extension requires only definitive surgery with adjuvant therapy.
C. Large-volume bilateral neck disease with extranodal extension favours chemoradiotherapy over surgery.
D. Levels IIA, III, and IV are dissected only in suspected cutaneous or nasopharyngeal SCC.
E. Bilateral palatine tonsillectomy is required if no primary is found.

Q15. A 55-year-old patient presents with a neck mass suspicious for malignancy. The clinical team is considering the appropriate preoperative evaluation. Which of the following is the most appropriate next step in the diagnostic workup for this patient?

A. Perform fine-needle aspiration or core biopsy of the suspicious neck mass.
B. Fibreoptic laryngoscopy is not required if contrast-enhanced CT of the neck has already been performed.
C. Perform PET-CT as the initial diagnostic test for metastatic cervical lymphadenopathy.
D. Perform high-risk HPV testing on all cervical lymph nodes.
E. Perform immediate MRI neck for all patients with neck lumps of unknown cause.

Q16. A 42-year-old male presents with a painless, slow-growing mass on the lateral neck. FNAC reveals spindle cells with no evidence of malignancy. What is the most likely diagnosis?

A. Pleomorphic adenoma
B. Lipoma
C. Schwannoma
D. Spindle Cell Carcinoma
E. Lymphangioma

Q17. A 62-year-old female presents with a red and white patch on the lateral border of her tongue. She has a history of 15 pack-years of smoking but denies alcohol use. A biopsy reveals abnormal superficial mitoses, increased mitotic figures, dyskeratosis, and nuclear pleomorphism extending into the middle third of the epithelium. Based on the WHO 2017 criteria, what is the most appropriate diagnosis?

A. Mild dysplasia
B. Moderate dysplasia
C. Severe dysplasia
D. Hyperkeratosis with no dysplasia
E. Carcinoma in situ

Q18. A 57-year-old male presents with a 3.5 cm ulcerated lesion on the right lateral border of the tongue. Biopsy confirms SCC. Imaging reveals invasion into the underlying tongue musculature with a depth of invasion (DOI) of 11 mm. There is a single ipsilateral lymph node measuring 3.5 cm, without ENE. No evidence of distant metastasis is found. Based on the TNM 8th edition staging, which of the following is the correct staging for this patient?

A. T2 N2a M0
B. T3 N2a M0
C. T2 N2b M0
D. T3 N1 M0
E. T4a N1 M1

Q19. A 55-year-old patient presents with a T2 tumour of the left buccal mucosa. Imaging and clinical examination show no evidence of cervical lymphadenopathy (N0). What is the most appropriate management of the neck in this patient?

A. Observation and regular follow-up
B. Elective neck dissection
C. Sentinel lymph node biopsy
D. Chemoradiotherapy
E. Radical neck dissection

Q20. A 62-year-old patient with SCC extending from the left palatine tonsils in the oropharynx to the retromolar region is being discussed at the multidisciplinary team (MDT) meeting. Biopsy results confirm SCC. HPV testing is positive. Which of the following statements is true?

A. Adjuvant radiotherapy is not recommended.
B. A histological margin of >2 cm is required.
C. Levels I–VI neck dissection is required.
D. HPV status will influence whether surgical or radical radiotherapy should be chosen.
E. HPV status affects prognosis.

Q21. A 55-year-old patient is diagnosed with a T1a SCC of the glottic larynx. According to current guidelines, what is the most appropriate initial management option?

A. Radiotherapy
B. Transoral laser microsurgery
C. Total laryngectomy
D. Chemoradiotherapy
E. Watchful waiting

Q22. A 60-year-old male presents with locally advanced squamous cell carcinoma (SCC) of the hypopharynx. After a multidisciplinary team (MDT) discussion, it is determined that he may be a candidate for larynx-preserving treatment, which includes radiation and either neoadjuvant or concomitant chemotherapy. According to current guidelines, which of the following factors would exclude this patient from larynx-preserving treatment?

A. Presence of cervical lymph node metastasis (N2b)
B. Recurrent aspiration pneumonias

C. Comorbidities such as uncontrolled diabetes mellitus and coronary artery disease
D. Tumour staging T2N0M0
E. Age greater than 70 years

Q23. A 76-year-old male presents to the Accident & Emergency (A&E) department with worsening breathing difficulties. He has a history of recurrent oral squamous cell carcinoma (SCC), which has rapidly progressed to involve the laryngopharynx. A recent CT scan shows distant bony metastasis. The patient's performance status is poor, and he is not a candidate for curative treatment. What is the most appropriate management to palliate his breathing difficulties?
A. Tracheostomy to secure the airway
B. Chemoradiotherapy to reduce tumour size
C. Endoluminal debulking of the tumour
D. Palliative radiotherapy to reduce tumour size
E. Palliative care referral without further intervention

Q24. A 64-year-old male is undergoing a left neck dissection for the management of T2N1M0 squamous cell carcinoma of the tongue. During the procedure, there is intraoperative suspicion of a thoracic duct injury. Which of the following statements is true regarding the management of a chyle leak?
A. A high-fat diet should be initiated to reduce chyle flow.
B. Trendelenburg position will help confirm successful management.
C. Octreotide is contraindicated in patients with high-volume chyle leaks.
D. Transabdominal thoracic duct embolisation (TDE) is the first-line surgical approach.
E. Orlistat is the preferred first-line conservative treatment.

Q25. A 52-year-old man of southern Chinese descent presents with a 2-month history of nasal obstruction, recurrent epistaxis, and left-sided hearing loss. He reports a growing left-sided neck mass. Examination reveals bilateral cervical lymphadenopathy and cranial nerve VI palsy. Imaging confirms a mass in the nasopharynx with involvement of the skull base. Biopsy confirms non-keratinising nasopharyngeal carcinoma (NPC). Which of the following is the most appropriate management plan for this patient?
A. Radiotherapy alone to the primary site and cervical lymph nodes
B. Concurrent chemoradiotherapy (CRT) with intensity-modulated radiotherapy (IMRT)
C. Primary surgery with endoscopic transnasal resection followed by radiotherapy
D. Neoadjuvant chemotherapy followed by surgery and radiotherapy
E. Observation and follow-up for disease progression

Q26. A 63-year-old woman undergoes wide local excision of a T2 oral squamous cell carcinoma (OSCC) of the tongue with simultaneous selective neck dissection (SND). The pathological report reveals clear margins of 3 mm, no extracapsular spread (ECS), and one positive lymph node. Which of the following statements is correct?
A. A pathological margin of 3 mm is considered close and requires re-resection.
B. Frozen section analysis during surgery is the standard of care for all T1/T2 OSCC cases.

C. Postoperative radiotherapy is indicated for patients with pathological margins <5 mm.
D. Elective neck dissection is unnecessary for patients with clinically N0 neck and T1/T2 tumours.
E. Elective neck dissection reveals occult metastasis in over 25% of T1/T2 OSCC cases with clinically N0 neck.

Q27. A 55-year-old patient recently diagnosed with a T3 tumour of the oropharynx is complaining of intractable ear pain. Which of the following is the most likely explanation?
A. Referred pain via the great auricular nerve
B. Referred pain via the auriculotemporal nerve
C. Referred pain via the lesser occipital nerve
D. Referred pain via the auricular branch of the vagus nerve
E. Referred pain via the facial nerve

Q28. A 55-year-old male presents with a non-healing leukoplakic lesion on the lateral border of his tongue. A Lugol's iodine stain is applied to assess the extent of dysplasia. What is the expected reaction of the dysplastic epithelium to Lugol's iodine?
A. Uniform dark brown staining
B. Patchy or absent staining
C. Bright yellow fluorescence under UV light
D. Blue-black discoloration
E. Green staining with methylene blue counterstain

ANSWERS AND EXPLANATIONS

Q1. **Dysplasia**

Answer: B. Loss of polarity of basal cells

Explanation: The WHO criteria for epithelial dysplasia include both architectural and cellular changes. "Loss of polarity of basal cells" is a hallmark feature under the architectural changes category, reflecting disorganised alignment of basal cells with respect to the basement membrane.

A. Uniform epithelial stratification with orderly nuclear arrangement: This describes normal epithelial tissue, not dysplasia. Dysplastic tissue shows irregular stratification.
B. Absence of mitotic figures in all epithelial layers: Dysplastic epithelium typically exhibits an *increased number of mitotic figures*, including in superficial layers, which is abnormal.
C. Uniform nuclear size and shape (no pleomorphism): Dysplastic cells display nuclear pleomorphism, including abnormal variation in nuclear size and shape.
D. Increased cellular cohesion with no keratinisation: Dysplastic epithelium often shows *loss of epithelial cell cohesion* and premature keratinisation (dyskeratosis).

Q2. **Adjuvant radiotherapy**

Answer: C. Nodal metastasis with extranodal extension

Explanation: ENE is a high-risk feature that strongly predicts the need for adjuvant radiotherapy due to its association with poor prognosis and increased recurrence risk. postoperative radiotherapy is recommended if close margins (<2 mm), extracapsular spread (ECS), multiple positive nodes, perineural invasion (PNI), or lymphovascular invasion (LVI).

Q3. **Lymph node metastasis**

Answer: D. Cystic degeneration of a lymph node metastasis

Explanation: In older patients, a cystic neck lump is most often due to metastatic disease, particularly from SCC. The brown aspirate suggests haemorrhagic or necrotic changes, commonly seen in cystic degeneration of metastatic nodes. Branchial cleft cysts and thyroglossal duct cysts are more common in younger patients. Papillary thyroid carcinoma cystic metastases are typically located in the central compartment. Parathyroid adenomas are solid, not cystic.

Q4. **HPV status**

Answer: B. Improves prognosis due to better response to treatment

Explanation: HPV-positive oropharyngeal cancers have better outcomes due to enhanced response to radiotherapy and chemotherapy compared to HPV-negative cancers. Patients are often younger, and HPV-negative cases are more likely to be associated with smoking and alcohol. As a result, the five-year survival rate for advanced-stage HPV-positive OPSCC is 75%–80%, compared to less than 50% for HPV-negative tumours. HPV oncogenes (*E6* and *E7*) act as key drivers of pathogenesis and may be important in the development of targeted therapies.

Q5. **Chemotherapy agents**

Answer: B. Cetuximab acts by targeting the extracellular domain of EGFR and may cause acneiform skin rash.

Explanation: Cisplatin works by forming DNA cross-links that disrupt DNA synthesis with toxicities including nephrotoxicity, ototoxicity, nausea, peripheral neuropathy, hepatotoxicity, and bone marrow suppression. Cetuximab is a monoclonal antibody targeting the extracellular domain of EGFR, inhibiting oncogenic signalling; it commonly causes an acneiform rash, often linked to better outcomes, as well as hypomagnesaemia. In contrast, 5-fluorouracil (5-FU) is an antimetabolite that inhibits thymidylate synthase to impair RNA synthesis, with side effects such as bone marrow suppression, diarrhoea, and cardiotoxicity. Cetuximab is an alternative to cisplatin for patients who cannot tolerate it but does not show superior efficacy in all HNSCC treatment settings.

Q6. **Types of thyroid carcinoma**

Answer: A. Papillary thyroid carcinoma

Explanation: Papillary thyroid carcinoma (PTC) is the most common type of thyroid malignancy, characterised by excellent prognosis and unique histological features. The presence of nuclear grooves and "Orphan Annie eye" nuclei, caused by chromatin clearing, are hallmark findings on cytology, distinguishing PTC from other thyroid lesions. Follicular thyroid carcinoma, while less common, tends to spread haematogenously and lacks the nuclear features of PTC. Medullary thyroid carcinoma arises from parafollicular C cells and is associated with calcitonin secretion, often linked to genetic syndromes like MEN2. Anaplastic thyroid carcinoma is an aggressive, undifferentiated tumour with poor prognosis, while thyroid adenomas are benign and lack malignant features.

Q7. **Management of thyroid malignancy**

Answer: B. Total thyroidectomy

Explanation: Hypoechoic lesions with microcalcifications on ultrasound are highly suspicious for malignancy and the histology suggests follicular thyroid carcinoma. FNAC confirming malignancy warrants total thyroidectomy in most cases, depending on the stage and type of cancer.

Q8. **Segmental mandibulectomy**

Answer: C. Segmental mandibulectomy

Explanation: Marginal mandibulectomy involves resecting part of the height of the mandible with resultant preservation of the continuity of the mandible. Segmental mandibulectomy involves resection of the entire vertical height of the mandible with interruption of the continuity of the mandible. Limited evidence for five-year survival outcome in literature but tendency in favour of segmental mandibulectomy was confirmed when medullary invasion was evident. As a result, segmental mandibulectomy is chosen when cortical bone destruction is evident to ensure oncologic clearance.

Q9. **Sentinel lymph node biopsy**

Answer: C. Sentinel lymph node biopsy (SLNB)

Explanation: According to NICE guidance, SLNB should be offered or discussed with patients who have melanoma with Breslow thickness ranging from 0.8 mm to 1 mm without ulceration, or less than 1 mm but with ulceration (classified as PT1b). This includes patients with stage I–II melanoma (AJCC staging, with stages IB–IIC). In the case of clinically N0 patients with melanoma, SLNB is a valuable procedure to assess for micrometastasis in the regional lymph nodes, which can guide further management. Elective neck dissection or postoperative adjuvant radiotherapy is not typically recommended unless lymph node involvement is detected, or the patient's condition worsens. Observation is appropriate only if the SLNB is negative, and no further intervention is needed.

Q10. **Investigation for squamous cell carcinoma of unknown primary**

Answer: B. Ipsilateral palatine tonsillectomy with or without lingual tonsillectomy

Explanation: For patients with unilateral SCCUP and no identified primary on initial evaluation, ipsilateral palatine tonsillectomy should be performed. If the primary is not found after this, lingual tonsillectomy may be considered. In cases where the primary remains undetected, additional surgical procedures may be required to identify the site of origin. Random biopsies of nonsuspicious areas have a low yield and are not recommended.

Q11. **Neck management for squamous cell carcinoma of unknown primary**

Answer: B. Neck dissection of levels IIA, III, and IV

Explanation: For SCCUP, levels IIA, III, and IV should be routinely dissected if an oropharyngeal primary is suspected. The extent of neck dissection should be based on the location of the metastatic lymph nodes. Bilateral neck dissection may be required in cases of bilateral involvement, but dissection should be tailored to the patient's specific presentation and multidisciplinary discussion. Radiotherapy may be considered in certain cases but typically follows after surgical evaluation.

Q12. **Management of leucoplakia**

Answer: B. Surgical excision of the lesion

Explanation: Severe dysplasia within a leukoplakic lesion is a high-risk precursor to invasive carcinoma and requires surgical excision to prevent malignant transformation. Simple observation is inadequate given the dysplastic changes. While laser ablation is an option for some lesions, surgical excision is preferred for better histopathological evaluation. Radiotherapy and topical steroids are not indicated for managing dysplasia.

Q13. **Radiotherapy for squamous cell carcinoma of unknown primary**

Answer: A. Radiotherapy targeting the bilateral neck nodes and mucosal regions at risk

Explanation: For patients with bilateral SCCUP, radiotherapy should target not only the gross disease in the neck but also the mucosal regions at risk of harbouring the occult primary tumour, including the oropharynx and other mucosal sites. The treatment volumes are based on clinicopathologic evaluation, and concurrent chemotherapy may be considered, especially for HPV-negative SCC. Chemotherapy alone or observation without treatment are not recommended for SCCUP without a known primary tumour (1).

Q14. **Neck management for squamous cell carcinoma of unknown primary**

Answer: C. Large-volume bilateral neck disease with extranodal extension favours chemoradiotherapy over surgery.

Explanation: Large-volume bilateral neck disease with ENE is best managed with definitive chemoradiotherapy, as it reduces the morbidity associated with extensive bilateral neck dissection while providing effective control of the disease. For unilateral, small-volume neck disease, both surgery and radiotherapy are valid options after multidisciplinary discussion. In cases of bilateral neck disease without ENE, treatment options include surgery with or without adjuvant therapy or radiotherapy with or without chemotherapy. Dissection of levels IIA, III, and IV is typically indicated for suspected oropharyngeal SCC, not limited to cutaneous or nasopharyngeal SCC. Bilateral palatine tonsillectomy is not universally required in SCCUP cases but is guided by clinical suspicion and diagnostic findings (1).

Q15. **Fine-needle aspiration and core biopsy**

Answer: A. Perform fine-needle aspiration or core biopsy of the suspicious neck mass

Explanation: Fine-needle aspiration or core biopsy is strongly recommended for a suspicious neck mass. This step is essential for obtaining a histopathologic diagnosis, which can guide further management. Contrast-enhanced CT (CECT) is typically used after biopsy for imaging, and fibreoptic laryngoscopy is recommended to identify a primary tumour. PET-CT is generally used when a primary tumour is not found on clinical examination or CECT. High-risk HPV testing is routinely done for SCCUP nodes at levels II and III but is not required for all lymph nodes.

Q16. **Benign neck lumps**

Answer: C. Schwannoma

Explanation: Schwannomas are benign nerve sheath tumours often presenting as painless, slow-growing masses in the head and neck. They are commonly associated with spindle cells on FNAC. Spindle cell carcinomas are aggressive variants of SCC and can be difficult to diagnose because its spindle cell component can mimic other lesions. As the stem states no evidence of malignancy, then carcinoma can be excluded.

Q17. **Dysplasia**

Answer: B. Moderate dysplasia

Explanation: The WHO 2017 classification of epithelial dysplasia categorises the severity of dysplasia based on the extent of histological abnormalities:

Mild dysplasia: Changes confined to the upper third of the epithelium.

Moderate dysplasia: Changes extend into the middle third of the epithelium (as seen in this case).

Severe dysplasia: Changes affect more than two-thirds of the epithelium, possibly including the full thickness.

Carcinoma in situ (E): This term was in the 2005 classification but removed in the WHO 2017 changes. It is now considered synonymous with severe dysplasia, making it redundant. In the WHO 2017 system, severe dysplasia includes cases previously labelled as carcinoma in situ.

Q18. **TNM classification (8th edition)**

Answer: B. T3 N2a M0

Explanation: Based on TNM 8th edition (see the following) applied to this example

Tumour (T): The lesion is **3.5 cm**, falling into **T2** based on size. However, the DOI is **11 mm**, upgrading it to **T3**.

Node (N): A single ipsilateral lymph node is **3.5 cm** and ENE-negative, corresponding to **N2a**.

Metastasis (M): No distant metastasis is evident, making this **M0**.

TNM 8th Edition Staging Criteria

T Category (Tumour)

TX: Primary tumour cannot be assessed.

Tis: Carcinoma in situ.

T1: Tumour ≤2 cm in greatest dimension and DOI ≤5 mm.

T2: Tumour >2 cm but ≤4 cm, or DOI >5 mm but ≤10 mm.

T3: Tumour >4 cm in size, or DOI >10 mm.

T4: Moderately or very advanced local disease:

T4a: Tumour invades adjacent structures like cortical bone, inferior alveolar nerve, maxillary sinus, or skin of face. For oral cavity tumours, superficial bone erosion alone (e.g., by a gingival tumour) is insufficient to classify as T4.

T4b: Very advanced disease, involving the masticator space, pterygoid plates, skull base, or encasing the internal carotid artery.

N Category (Nodal)

NX: Regional lymph nodes cannot be assessed.

N0: No regional lymph node metastasis.

N1: Single ipsilateral lymph node metastasis, ≤3 cm in size, ENE-negative.

N2: Classified further into subcategories:

N2a: Single ipsilateral lymph node, >3 cm but ≤6 cm, ENE-negative.
N2b: Multiple ipsilateral lymph nodes, ≤6 cm, ENE-negative.
N2c: Bilateral or contralateral lymph nodes, ≤6 cm, ENE-negative.
N3: Advanced nodal disease:
N3a: Any lymph node >6 cm, ENE-negative.
N3b: Any node (s) with ENE-positive.
M Category (Metastasis)
M0: No evidence of distant metastasis.
M1: Evidence of distant metastasis.

Key Updates in TNM 8th Edition:

DOI: A critical factor for staging oral cavity cancers, incorporated into T1, T2, and T3 definitions.

Extranodal Extension (ENE): The presence of ENE now directly influences nodal staging, with ENE-positive nodes classified as N3b regardless of size.

Metastasis (M Category): M1 reflects distant metastatic spread, which is vital for prognosis and treatment decisions (2).

Q19. **Sentinel lymph node biopsy**

Answer: B. Elective neck dissection

Explanation: According to NICE Guideline 36 (2016) for managing early oral cavity cancer (T1–T2, N0):

SLNB is preferred over elective neck dissection for patients with early oral cavity cancer (T1–T2, N0), provided they do not require cervical access for other procedures (e.g., free-flap reconstruction).

SLNB effectively identifies occult nodal metastases while reducing surgical morbidity compared to elective neck dissection.

Elective neck dissection (B) may be considered if SLNB is not feasible or if cervical access is required for other surgical interventions.

Q20. **HPV status**

Answer: E. HPV status affects prognosis

Explanation: HPV status is a critical prognostic factor in oropharyngeal SCC. HPV-positive SCC is associated with better overall survival and treatment response compared to HPV-negative disease. This influences prognosis but does not directly determine whether surgery or radiotherapy is chosen, as the treatment strategy depends on tumour staging, patient factors, and multidisciplinary team (MDT) recommendations. Adjuvant radiotherapy is often indicated for advanced tumours or where surgical margins are close/positive or nodal involvement is significant. A clear surgical margin of ≥5 mm histologically is desired, and as a result, 1 cm clinical margins are aimed for.

Q21. **Management of laryngeal malignancy**

Answer: B. Transoral laser microsurgery

Explanation: For patients with newly diagnosed T1a SCC of the glottic larynx, transoral laser microsurgery is the recommended treatment per NICE guidelines. It is minimally invasive, preserves laryngeal function, and provides excellent oncologic outcomes for early stage disease. NICE recommends offering a choice of transoral laser microsurgery or radiotherapy to people with newly diagnosed T1b–T2 SCC of the glottic larynx (3).

Q22. **Management of laryngeal malignancy**

Answer: B. Recurrent aspiration pneumonias

Explanation: According to current NICE guidelines (3), larynx-preserving treatment for locally advanced SCC of the hypopharynx, which involves radiation and potentially neoadjuvant or concomitant chemotherapy, can be offered to patients if suitable and they do not have the following:

- Tumour-related dysphagia needing a feeding tube
- A compromised airway
- Recurrent aspiration pneumonias.

Q23. **Palliative management of breathlessness**

Answer: C. Endoluminal debulking of the tumour

Explanation: In this scenario, the patient has advanced recurrent oral SCC with airway obstruction due to tumour involvement in the laryngopharynx and distant bony metastasis. The most appropriate approach to palliate his breathing difficulties is endoluminal debulking. This procedure involves removing or reducing the tumour from within the airway to alleviate obstruction and improve respiratory function. It is preferred over a tracheostomy, when possible, as it avoids creating a permanent stoma and can provide symptom relief while maintaining some degree of normal airway function (3).

Q24. **Chyle leak**

Answer: B. Trendelenburg position will help confirm successful management.

Explanation: Management of thoracic duct injury involves both conservative and surgical approaches depending on the severity of the leak. If noticed intraoperatively, ligation of the open duct is the most effective way to stop chyle leak. A variety of techniques have been described in the literature including suturing, clipping, fibrin glues and local sclerosing agents. Many advocate the covering of the repaired lesion with an additional muscle layer—e.g., SCM. Delay of enteral feeding for patients with intraoperatively recognised chyle leak is recommended. Post repair Valsalva manoeuvre and Trendelenburg position help to identify ongoing leak. A low-fat diet rich in medium-chain triglycerides (MCTs) is a first-line conservative measure to reduce chyle production. Octreotide is a somatostatin analogue which reduces the production of lymphatic contents by inhibiting the production of pancreatic and gastrointestinal enzymes. It is most effective for low volume leaks but is of benefit even in high-volume leaks (>100 ml/day) with prolonged treatment, though it should be used cautiously in patients with cardiovascular or hepatic conditions. TDE is a second-line surgical option after failure of local measures. Orlistat inactivates pancreatic enzymes and prevents the resorption of fat cells in the intestine, and their entry into the enteral circulation. It is a second-line option.

Q25. **Nasopharyngeal carcinoma**

Answer: B. Concurrent chemoradiotherapy (CRT) with intensity-modulated radiotherapy (IMRT).

Explanation: This patient has advanced-stage NPC involving the skull base and cervical lymph nodes (stage III/IV). CRT with IMRT is the gold standard treatment for advanced NPC, as it improves overall survival and disease control in stage III/IV disease. IMRT optimally targets the tumour while sparing surrounding tissues. While radiotherapy is effective for early stage disease (stage I/II), CRT is superior in advanced-stage NPC. Surgery is not the primary treatment for NPC due to the location and is typically reserved for residual or recurrent disease. Observation is inappropriate for symptomatic advanced-stage NPC with significant morbidity and risk of progression.

Q26. **Elective neck dissection N0 neck**

Answer: E. Elective neck dissection reveals occult metastasis in over 25% of T1/T2 OSCC cases with clinically N0 neck.

Explanation: Elective neck dissection or sentinel node biopsy is strongly recommended for T1/T2 OSCC with a clinically N0 neck due to the high incidence of occult metastasis, as demonstrated by the D'Cruz study (2015), where 29.6% of patients had occult nodal involvement identified through elective neck dissection. Evidence around margins and recurrence is controversial and pathological margins as close as 2 mm may provide good local control. Therefore, they do not typically require re-resection unless other high-risk features (e.g., PNI or LVI) are present. Similarly postoperative radiotherapy is recommended if close margins (<2 mm), extracapsular spread (ECS), multiple positive nodes, PNI, or LVI. Frozen sections are useful in recurrent or complex cases but are not standard for all T1/T2 OSCC surgeries (4).

Q27. **Anatomy of the vagus nerve**

Answer: D. Referred pain via the auricular branch of the vagus nerve

Explanation: Patients with oropharyngeal tumours may experience referred ear pain due to the shared innervation between the oropharynx and the ear through the auricular branch of the vagus nerve. This branch provides sensation to the concha and posterior auditory canal, and oropharyngeal cancers, such as those involving the tonsil, base of tongue, or soft palate, can cause referred pain in this region. This pathway is distinct to the vagus nerve and not associated with the great auricular, auriculotemporal, or lesser occipital, which innervate other areas of the ear.

Q28. **Lugol's iodine test**

Answer: B. Patchy or absent staining

Explanation: Lugol's iodine selectively stains normal oral mucosa dark brown due to its high glycogen content, as iodine binds to glycogen molecules. Dysplastic or precancerous tissue, however, has reduced or absent glycogen levels due to altered cellular metabolism, preventing iodine uptake and resulting in a pale or unstained appearance. This contrast allows clinicians to visually identify suspicious areas for biopsy and further evaluation. A positive Lugol's iodine reaction (dark-brown staining) indicates healthy tissue, whereas a negative reaction (pale or unstained areas) suggests potential dysplasia. Other options listed, such as bright yellow fluorescence (C) or blue-black discoloration (D), are associated with different diagnostic techniques unrelated to glycogen staining.

2 Head and Neck Reconstructive Surgery

QUESTIONS

Q1. A 78-year-old patient is undergoing excision and reconstruction of a lip SCC. Which of the following statements is correct?

A. The Abbe flap is a fan-shaped rotational flap used for large lower lip defects involving more than 50% of the lip.
B. The Estlander flap is based on the superior labial artery and is designed for lateral lower lip defects involving the commissure.
C. The Gillies fan flap is a triangular flap based on the inferior labial artery, typically used for upper lip reconstruction.
D. The McGregor flap reduces the size of the oral stoma when rotated around the commissure.
E. The Karapandzic flap requires a secondary mucosal advancement flap for lip mucosa reconstruction.

Q2. One of your colleagues has proposed using a jejunal flap. Which of the following statements about its use for intraoral reconstruction is correct?

A. The jejunum flap is unsuitable for microsurgical anastomoses due to the unreliability of its vascular pedicle.
B. Jejunal flaps are best suited for reconstructing tongue and floor-of-mouth (FOM) defects as they allow full tongue mobility and provide a secretory lining.
C. The jejunum flap lacks secretory function and is therefore unsuitable for preventing xerostomia in irradiated patients.
D. The blood supply to the jejunum flap is provided by branches of the inferior mesenteric artery.
E. Bowel continuity is reestablished as a delayed procedure after loop ileostomy.

Q3. A 50-year-old patient with a history of facial paralysis undergoes electromyography (EMG) testing, which shows partial denervation of the facial muscles, with weak but present movement on the affected side. Which of the following is the most appropriate reanimation strategy?

A. Direct nerve repair
B. Myocutaneous free flap reconstruction
C. Cross-facial nerve grafting (CFNG) to supplement existing movement without disrupting residual function
D. Free muscle transfer without nerve input
E. Immediate full muscle substitution

DOI: 10.1201/9781003609308-3

Q4. During the harvest of a radial forearm free flap under tourniquet control, careful dissection is performed along the forearm. To preserve flap viability and minimise sensory or functional deficits, which of the following anatomical guidelines is most crucial to follow?

A. The dissection should proceed proximally only as far as the radial artery's bifurcation from the brachial artery to avoid sacrificing the radial recurrent artery.
B. Dissection should remain in the supramuscular plane to avoid damaging the paratenon of the underlying flexor carpi radialis.
C. The radial artery should be mobilised carefully between the flexor carpi radialis and the brachioradialis muscles along the lateral aspect of the forearm.
D. The superficial palmar arch must be dissected and ligated to prevent ischaemia to the thumb and index finger.
E. The flap should be raised without tourniquet use to preserve the vascular integrity of the flexor pollicis longus.

Q5. When harvesting an osseocutaneous radial forearm free flap (OCRFFF) for mandibular reconstruction, prophylactic internal fixation (PIF) of the radius is often employed. Which of the following statements best reflects the rationale for selective use of PIF in this procedure?

A. PIF allows up to 70% of the radial circumference to be harvested without risk of fracture.
B. The use of PIF has been shown to reduce the risk of postoperative radial fractures to below 5% in all patients.
C. Older females with osteopenia and smaller radial diameter are at increased risk of fracture without PIF.
D. Distal osteotomy should be within 1 cm of the radial styloid to maximise the length of bone harvest.
E. Postoperative immobilisation with a below-elbow cast for three weeks is sufficient to prevent fracture in all patients.

Q6. A 60-year-old man undergoes radial forearm free flap (RFFF) harvest for intraoral reconstruction. Three months later, he presents with persistent numbness over the dorsoradial aspect of his hand and reduced grip strength. His range of wrist motion has decreased slightly compared to preoperative levels. What is the most appropriate management strategy for his symptoms?

A. Observation and reassurance, as sensory and strength deficits will resolve without intervention
B. Immediate referral for surgical decompression of the radial nerve
C. Physiotherapy to improve strength and range of motion
D. Exploration and grafting of the ulnar nerve
E. Application of a wrist splint to improve strength

Q7. A 52-year-old man with a history of smoking and type 2 diabetes undergoes fibular free flap harvest for mandibular reconstruction. One week postoperatively, he develops a partial skin graft loss and wound dehiscence at the donor site. What is the most appropriate management strategy to promote wound healing and facilitate earlier mobilisation?

A. Revision surgery with repeat split-thickness skin grafting
B. Application of negative pressure wound therapy (NPWT)
C. Daily dressing changes with saline-moistened gauze
D. Debridement and primary closure of the wound
E. Below-knee casting to protect the wound

Q8. A 47-year-old woman develops stiffness and "clawing" of the great toe following fibular free flap harvest for mandibular reconstruction. Which of the following is the most likely cause of this complication?
A. Injury to the peroneal nerve
B. Dissection extending too proximally near the fibular head
C. Detachment or injury to the flexor hallucis longus muscle
D. Harvest of excessive fibular bone leading to ankle instability
E. Compression of the superficial peroneal nerve in the lateral compartment

Q9. A 54-year-old man undergoes an anterolateral thigh (ALT) free flap for head and neck reconstruction. One month postoperatively, he reports numbness over a large area on his thigh. Which of the following best explains this complication?
A. Injury to the superficial femoral nerve
B. Harvesting a wide skin paddle including the lateral femoral cutaneous nerve
C. Transection of the femoral nerve motor branches
D. Damage to the descending branch of the lateral circumflex femoral artery
E. Compression of the sciatic nerve

Q10. A 62-year-old man undergoes scapula free flap harvest for reconstruction of a mandibular defect. Two months postoperatively, he reports shoulder weakness and reduced shoulder mobility. Which of the following is the most likely cause of his symptoms?
A. Injury to the circumflex scapular nerve
B. Fracture of the scapular body
C. Shoulder joint dislocation
D. Detachment of the rotator cuff
E. Expected harvest-related reduction in shoulder strength and range of motion

Q11. During the harvest of a scapular free flap with an osteocutaneous component, a surgeon plans to harvest a segment of the lateral scapular border. Which of the following steps is crucial to preserving the shoulder function and vascular integrity of surrounding structures?
A. Dividing the teres minor muscle to improve access to the circumflex scapular artery
B. Harvesting the bone segment from 2 cm below the glenohumeral joint to the scapular spine
C. Carefully detaching and potentially reattaching the teres major and long head of the triceps to the scapula
D. Reflecting the subscapularis muscle to expose the lateral scapular border
E. Avoiding release of the infraspinatus muscle from the scapular spine

Q12. A 58-year-old man undergoes mandibular reconstruction using a deep circumflex iliac artery (DCIA) free flap with an internal oblique muscle component. Two weeks postoperatively, he develops swelling at the donor site. An ultrasound shows a fluid collection. There are no signs or symptoms of infection. The area is fluctuant with normal overlying skin and no bruising. What is the most appropriate initial management of this complication?

A. Open surgical drainage of the donor site
B. Application of negative pressure wound therapy
C. Needle aspiration with repeated aspirations as necessary
D. Placement of a surgical drain and reoperation
E. Compression bandaging to reduce swelling

Q13. A 62-year-old woman undergoes mandibular reconstruction with a DCIA free flap. Closure of the donor site required mesh to replace the defect. Three weeks postoperatively, she reports worsening pain at the donor site and signs of wound infection. She is admitted by the on-call team and receives 48 hours of IV antibiotics. Ultrasound shows a drainable collection. What is the most appropriate next step in management?

A. Switch to oral antibiotics and monitor
B. Perform incision and drainage under local anaesthetic
C. Apply negative pressure wound therapy to manage the infection
D. Increase immobilisation with a supportive abdominal binder
E. Perform surgical debridement and remove the mesh

Q14. You assess a 70-year-old woman pre-operatively who is scheduled for mandibular reconstruction after resection of an oral malignancy which extends into the mandible. She has been consented by the registrar for a DCIA flap. Her medical history includes obesity (BMI 41), chronic gait instability, a repaired inguinal hernia, and prior surgery on her left iliac crest for bone graft harvest. Additionally, she recently underwent radiation therapy to the head and neck. Which of the following would be the most appropriate next step?

A. Proceed with DCIA flap harvest despite her prior iliac crest surgery
B. Use a scapula free flap instead
C. Perform a thorough preoperative CT angiogram to evaluate the patency of the iliac vessels
D. Proceed with DCIA flap harvest but limit the bone harvest to avoid weakening the iliac crest
E. Use a myocutaneous radial forearm flap instead

Q15. A 52-year-old patient requires a trapezius flap for reconstruction following extensive excision of a soft tissue sarcoma on the neck. Which artery primarily supplies the trapezius flap?

A. Transverse cervical artery
B. Suprascapular artery
C. Thoracoacromial artery
D. Subclavian artery
E. Brachial artery

Q16. A 63-year-old patient undergoes excision of an advanced head and neck tumour, requiring reconstruction with a deltopectoral flap. What is the main arterial supply to this flap?

A. Internal mammary artery
B. Thoracoacromial artery
C. Lateral thoracic artery
D. Transverse cervical artery
E. Subclavian artery

Q17. A 68-year-old patient undergoes excision of a biopsy-proven nodular basal cell carcinoma on the nasal tip. The defect is 2 cm in diameter and involves the nasal cartilage. What is the most appropriate reconstructive option?

A. Full-thickness skin graft from the supraclavicular area
B. Local advancement flap using nasolabial tissue
C. Paramedian forehead flap
D. Delayed healing with secondary intention
E. Split-thickness skin graft

Q18. A 35-year-old patient underwent enucleation of a large odontogenic keratocyst in the left mandible, leaving a substantial bony defect. What is the most appropriate reconstructive option in this case?

A. Immediate free vascularised fibula graft
B. Immediate placement of autologous cancellous bone graft
C. Allow healing by secondary intention with periodic follow-up
D. Reconstruction with titanium implant and bone grafting after healing
E. Delayed reconstruction with particulate bone graft after healing

Q19. A 67-year-old patient underwent a paramedian forehead flap for nasal reconstruction following excision of a basal cell carcinoma. On postoperative day 2, the flap appears dusky and congested. What is the most appropriate initial step in management?

A. Immediate return to theatre for flap revision
B. Apply leeches to the flap
C. Administer intravenous heparin
D. Inspect and release tension sutures at the base of the flap
E. Make no changes and continue regular observation

Q20. A 54-year-old patient who underwent reconstruction with a radial forearm free flap reports significant pain and discoloration of their thumb and all fingers postoperatively. What is the most likely cause?

A. Inadequate flap perfusion
B. Injury to the ulnar artery during surgery
C. Thrombosis in the radial artery
D. Venous thrombosis
E. Vasospasm of the palmar arches

Q21. A 40-year-old patient undergoes neck dissection for parotid malignancy. During surgery, a vein is identified descending within the gland and lying deep to the branches of the facial nerve. Which of the following is true regarding this vein?

A. It drains directly into the internal jugular vein
B. It is formed by the union of the maxillary vein and superficial temporal vein
C. It is formed from the posterior retromandibular vein and posterior auricular vein
D. It crosses superficial to the sternocleidomastoid muscle to reach the subclavian vein
E. It is a tributary of the facial vein

Q22. During a neck dissection for a patient with metastatic lymphadenopathy, a vein is identified superficial to the investing layer of the deep cervical fascia. Which of the following is true regarding this vein?
A. It drains directly into the subclavian vein
B. It is formed by the union of the posterior retromandibular vein and the anterior jugular vein
C. It runs deep to the sternocleidomastoid muscle before joining the internal jugular vein
D. It is formed by the anterior retromandibular vein and posterior auricular vein
E. It passes through the carotid sheath

Q23. A 34-year-old male undergoes cheiloplasty for lower lip reconstruction after excision of a T1 squamous cell carcinoma. Which of the following techniques provides the best functional and aesthetic result for a defect involving 50% of the lower lip?
A. Karapandzic flap
B. Abbe flap
C. Estlander flap
D. Gillies fan flap
E. V-Y advancement flap

Q24. A 55-year-old male undergoes fibular free flap reconstruction for a mandibular defect. On postoperative day 2, the flap appears cool, pale, and Doppler signals are absent. What is the next best step?
A. Administer systemic anticoagulation
B. Return to theatre for exploration
C. Start hyperbaric oxygen therapy
D. Elevate the head of the bed and monitor
E. Perform ultrasound of the anastomosis

Q25. A 58-year-old male with a temporary tracheostomy day 12 post-OSCC resection and reconstruction is being evaluated for decannulation. Which of the following is the most important functional criterion for safe decannulation?
A. Normal arterial blood gases on room air
B. Absence of respiratory secretions
C. Ability to tolerate tracheostomy occlusion and clear secretions
D. Able to tolerate cuff down for >24 hours
E. Normal swallowing studies

Q26. A patient has had a size 8 cuffed tracheostomy in situ for two months. Poor emergence profile and high cuff pressures have been noted on prior ward rounds. You are called to the ward due to significant haemorrhage from the tracheostomy. Which of the following is the likely cause?

A. Internal jugular vein
B. Subclavian artery
C. Innominate artery
D. Superior thyroid artery
E. Ascending laryngeal artery

Q27. While raising a fibula free flap for mandibular reconstruction, you are unable to identify a perforator. What is the most appropriate next step?
A. Abandon the fibula flap and consider an alternative donor site
B. Raise a skin paddle based on the septocutaneous perforators
C. Proceed with fibula harvest without including a skin paddle
D. Perform intraoperative angiography to confirm vascular anatomy
E. Use a fasciocutaneous paddle based on musculocutaneous perforators

Q28. A 60-year-old male with a buccal squamous cell carcinoma is scheduled for resection and reconstruction using a left radial forearm free flap. During the preoperative evaluation, the Allen's test reveals inadequate collateral circulation through the ulnar artery. What should be the next step in managing this patient, considering the right wrist had a significant trauma in a cycling accident requiring ORIF?
A. Switch to a right radial forearm free flap
B. Switch to an anterolateral thigh free flap
C. Perform a Doppler ultrasound to reassess the radial artery and proceed with surgery as planned
D. Cancel the surgery and reconsider radiotherapy with the MDT
E. Delay the surgery and optimise collateral circulation with physiotherapy

Q29. A 50-year-old male is undergoing mandibular reconstruction using a fibular free flap after segmental mandibulectomy for squamous cell carcinoma. During the surgery, there are concerns about the adequacy of the fibular bone stock for the defect length. What is the most appropriate approach to optimise the reconstruction?
A. Perform bilateral fibular free flaps to increase the bone volume
B. Augment the fibular graft with an iliac crest bone graft
C. Use the fibula for soft tissue reconstruction only and switch to a scapular osteocutaneous free flap for bone
D. Proceed with a single fibular free flap and delay bone grafting for a secondary procedure
E. Harvest additional bone from the contralateral fibula for extended reconstruction

Q30. A 42-year-old patient undergoes a radial forearm free flap reconstruction for intraoral defect repair. At the donor site, a split-thickness skin graft (STSG) is planned for closure. Which of the following statements about STSGs is TRUE?
A. STSGs can be used to cover tendon at the radial forearm donor site.
B. STSGs can tolerate up to four days of ischaemia before inosculation begins.
C. The donor site for an STSG heals slowly and cannot be reused.
D. Thin STSGs are best suited for covering mechanically demanding areas like the soles of the feet.
E. STSGs provide superior aesthetic match compared to full-thickness skin grafts (FTSGs) in visible areas like the face.

Q31. 28-year-old female patient presents with total eyebrow loss following a traumatic injury. Examination reveals significant scarring and thinning of the skin in the eyebrow area. What is the most appropriate method for eyebrow reconstruction in this case?

A. Hair plug transplantation from the scalp
B. Hair strip grafts from the scalp
C. Pedicled scalp flap from the temporoparietal region
D. Synthetic eyebrow tattooing
E. Observation and follow-up with potential grafting after scar maturation

ANSWERS AND EXPLANATIONS

Q1. **Estlander flap**

Answer: B. The Estlander flap is based on the superior labial artery and is designed for lateral lower lip defects involving the commissure.

Explanation: The Estlander flap is a triangular flap used for lateral lower lip defects that involve the commissure. It is based on the superior labial artery and involves a 180° transposition from the upper lip to the lower lip. This procedure can result in a smaller oral stoma and an indistinct commissure, which may require further revision. The Abbe flap, on the other hand, is a V-shaped flap based on the inferior labial artery, primarily used for central upper lip defects. The Gillies fan flap is indeed used for large lower lip defects but is based on the superior labial artery, not the inferior labial artery, and does not have a triangular shape. The McGregor flap does not reduce the oral stoma size, as it is designed to rotate around the commissure without altering the oral aperture. Finally, the Karapandzic flap is a neurovascular advancement flap that does not require a secondary mucosal advancement flap.

Q2. **Jejunum flap**

Answer: B. Jejunal flaps are best suited for reconstructing tongue and FOM defects as they allow full tongue mobility and provide a secretory lining.

Explanation: The jejunum free flap is advantageous for intraoral reconstruction, particularly in irradiated patients, due to its retained secretory function, which helps prevent xerostomia. Its flexibility and ability to provide bulk and lining make it ideal for reconstructing defects in the tongue and floor of the mouth, supporting a full range of motion. The flap has a reliable vascular pedicle, which is typically supplied by branches of the superior mesenteric artery (not the inferior mesenteric artery), making it suitable for microsurgical anastomoses. After flap harvest, bowel continuity at the donor site is reestablished surgically.

Q3. **Cross-facial nerve grafting**

Answer: C. Cross-facial nerve grafting (CFNG) to supplement existing movement without disrupting residual function

Explanation: In cases of partial denervation with weak but residual facial movement, CFNG is a preferred strategy to provide additional motor input to the facial muscles without disrupting the existing movement. CFNG can support reinnervation without compromising the remaining nerve function, thus enhancing movement while preserving what remains. Direct repair would only be an option if both nerve stumps were intact, which is not applicable here. Free muscle transfer without nerve input or full muscle substitution would only be considered if there were total atrophy of the facial muscles and no residual function, which is not indicated in this case.

Q4. **Radial forearm free flap**

Answer: C. The radial artery should be mobilised carefully between the flexor carpi radialis and the brachioradialis muscles along the lateral aspect of the forearm.

Explanation: In radial forearm free flap harvest, it is essential to identify the radial artery as it courses between the flexor carpi radialis and brachioradialis muscles on the lateral forearm. Staying in the subfascial plane and respecting these muscle boundaries preserves essential structures, especially the palmaris longus and flexor carpi radialis tendons. Dissecting beyond the brachial artery bifurcation is generally unnecessary, and avoiding paratenon damage at the harvest site supports flap integration. While the superficial palmar arch may have anatomical variations, it is not typically dissected or ligated in this procedure. A tourniquet is commonly used to minimise blood loss and optimise visibility.

Q5. **Osseocutaneous radial forearm free flap**

Answer: C. Older females with osteopenia and smaller radial diameter are at increased risk of fracture without PIF.

Explanation: PIF is selectively recommended, particularly for patients at higher risk of radial fracture, such as older females with smaller radial diameter and osteopenia. Studies have shown that without PIF, the fracture rate is approximately 13%–25%. However, in a series of patients with PIF, only one fracture was reported in 167 cases (5). Proper positioning of the distal osteotomy (at least 2 cm proximal to the radial styloid) allows space for two screws, thus reducing the risk of compromising the wrist joint. Above-elbow splinting initially, followed by a below-elbow cast for six weeks, is typically required for adequate stabilisation post-surgery. Harvest of less than 40% of the diameter of the radius bone and harvest in a boat shaped fashion has been suggested to minimise the risk of fracture without PIF.

Q6. **Postoperative complications of radial forearm free flap**

Answer: C. Physiotherapy to improve strength and range of motion

Explanation: Postoperative numbness over the dorsoradial hand and mild reduction in grip strength and wrist motion are common complications following radial forearm free flap harvest. Physiotherapy is recommended to restore strength and range of motion, as these functional impairments typically improve over time, with many patients reaching preoperative levels by 24 months. Surgical interventions, such as nerve decompression, are unnecessary unless severe neuropathic pain or motor deficits are present. A wrist splint is not beneficial for improving strength in this setting.

Q7. **Postoperative complications of fibular free flap**

Answer: B. Application of negative pressure wound therapy (NPWT)

Explanation: NPWT has been shown to improve wound healing, reduce healing time, and enhance graft take for skin grafts at the fibular donor site. This approach is particularly beneficial in patients with risk factors for wound complications, such as smoking and diabetes. Repeat grafting may be necessary in some cases, but NPWT is the preferred initial approach, as it supports wound bed preparation and minimises the need for further surgery. Daily dressing changes can delay healing, and below-knee casting would not address the wound healing issue directly.

Q8. **Postoperative complications of fibular free flap**

Answer: C. Detachment or injury to the flexor hallucis longus muscle

Explanation: Stiffness and clawing of the great toe are commonly associated with injury or detachment of the flexor hallucis longus (FHL) muscle during fibular free flap harvest. The FHL originates from the posterior surface of the fibula, and its involvement in the flap can lead to scarring, contracture, and subsequent toe deformities. Protecting this muscle, particularly through careful perforator dissection, can reduce this risk. Injury to the peroneal nerve or harvesting excessive fibular bone does not typically cause toe clawing but may lead to sensory deficits, ankle instability, or foot drop.

Q9. **Postoperative complications of anterolateral thigh flap**

Answer: B. Harvesting a wide skin paddle, including the lateral femoral cutaneous nerve

Explanation: The lateral femoral cutaneous nerve, which supplies sensation to the inferolateral thigh, is often included in the skin paddle during ALT flap harvest. This typically results in postoperative numbness or paraesthesia in the lateral thigh area, especially when a wider skin paddle is taken. Damage to the femoral nerve or its motor branches would more likely result in muscle weakness rather than numbness in this distribution. The superficial femoral and sciatic nerves are not directly affected by ALT flap harvest.

Q10. **Postoperative complications of scapula free flap**

Answer: E. Expected harvest-related reduction in shoulder strength and range of motion

Explanation: The scapula free flap harvest often results in a temporary reduction in shoulder strength and range of motion, particularly for abduction, flexion, and external rotation. Studies show that most functional deficits, including reduced strength and mobility, tend to improve within six months. Fracture of the scapular body is a possible but less common complication, and joint dislocation or rotator cuff detachment is unlikely, as they are not typically affected by the flap harvest. The circumflex scapular artery is the largest terminal branch of the subscapular artery. Important nerves around the scapula include the suprascapular, dorsal scapular, and subscapular (upper and lower) nerves.

Q11. **Scapula free flap**

Answer: C. Carefully detaching and potentially reattaching the teres major and long head of the triceps to the scapula

Explanation: When harvesting an osteocutaneous scapular flap, detaching the teres major and long head of the triceps is necessary for access to the lateral scapular border. To preserve shoulder function, reattaching these muscles to the remaining scapula is essential, usually by suturing through drill holes in the residual bone. Teres minor is not typically divided during flap harvest; access is obtained by dividing the teres major. The standard harvest zone extends only 1 cm below the glenohumeral joint to preserve shoulder stability. Infraspinatus, not the subscapularis, is reflected for access to the osteotomy line and partial release may be necessary to achieve adequate exposure.

Q12. **Deep circumflex iliac artery free flap**

Answer: C. Needle aspiration with repeated aspirations as necessary

Explanation: Seroma formation is a known complication following DCIA flap harvest, often due to disruption of external iliac lymphatics. Needle aspiration is typically the first-line treatment for seromas, and repeated aspirations may be required until fluid accumulation subsides. Open drainage or reoperation is not usually necessary unless there is infection or persistent seroma that does not respond to conservative management. Compression bandaging is less effective for seromas in this region.

Q13. **Postoperative complications of deep circumflex iliac artery free flap**

Answer: E. Perform surgical debridement and remove the mesh

Explanation: Infections involving the internal oblique mesh at the DCIA donor site are challenging to treat due to biofilm formation on the mesh which is difficult for antimicrobials to penetrate. Initial management may include debridement and antibiotic therapy, but persistent infection often necessitates removing the mesh to fully resolve the issue. Topical antiseptic dressings and NPWT may support wound healing but are insufficient alone if the mesh is infected.

Q14. **Indications and contraindications to flap choice**

Answer: B. Use a scapula free flap instead due to her history of gait instability and prior iliac crest surgery

Explanation: This patient has multiple contraindications for a DCIA flap, including prior iliac crest surgery, obesity, and chronic gait instability, which may be exacerbated by further manipulation of the iliac crest. The scapula free flap avoids these issues and provides a viable alternative without affecting her gait. A CT angiogram would not address these primary contraindications, and limiting bone harvest would still risk exacerbating gait instability and may not provide enough material for the reconstruction.

Q15. **Trapezius flap**

Answer: A. Transverse cervical artery

Explanation: The trapezius flap is primarily supplied by the superficial branch of the transverse cervical artery (SCA), which is also known as the superficial cervical artery. This artery supplies the transverse (middle) part of the trapezius. The ascending (inferior) part of the trapezius is supplied by the dorsal scapular artery (DSA), which is the deep branch of the transverse cervical artery.

Q16. **Deltopectoral flap**

Answer: A. Internal mammary artery

Explanation: The deltopectoral flap is a fasciocutaneous flap based on the perforators of the internal mammary artery. The thoracoacromial artery supplies adjacent tissues, but it is not the main artery for this flap.

Q17. **Paramedian forehead flap**

Answer: C. Paramedian forehead flap

Explanation: Reconstruction of the nasal tip, particularly for larger defects involving cartilage, often requires a forehead flap. This provides both robust vascularity and tissue matching in terms of colour and thickness. Local flaps or grafts may be used for smaller defects, but they are less suitable for larger or complex reconstructions involving cartilage. Secondary intention healing is not appropriate for defects of this size and depth.

Q18. **Delayed reconstruction**

Answer: E. Delayed reconstruction with particulate bone graft after healing

Explanation: Large dental cysts such as odontogenic keratocysts often require enucleation and curettage, leaving substantial bony defects. Immediate reconstruction is generally avoided due to the risk of recurrence or infection. Healing by secondary intention is typically allowed for 6–12 months, during which time there is usually some degree of bony infill. Subsequently, reconstruction can be performed using bone grafts or other appropriate techniques.

Q19. **Flap congestion**

Answer: D. Inspect and release tension sutures at the base of the flap

Explanation: A congested forehead flap often results from venous outflow obstruction. There may be a variety of causes, including excessive tension at the flap's pedicle. The first step is to inspect and release tension sutures or other factors causing compression. If venous congestion persists, then returning to theatre to identify and address the cause would be the likely next best step. If nothing is done, then congestion is likely to worsen, compromising the flap's viability.

Q20. **Postoperative complications of radial forearm free flap**

Answer: B. Injury to the ulnar artery during surgery

Explanation: When harvesting a radial forearm free flap, care must be taken to ensure adequate collateral blood flow via the ulnar artery to perfuse the hand. Preoperative Allen's test or other vascular assessments are critical to confirm ulnar artery patency. If the radial artery is harvested without sufficient collateral circulation, ischaemia of the thumb and index finger can occur. Venous thrombosis or inadequate flap perfusion would primarily affect the flap itself, not the hand. Vasospasm of the palmar arches is a rare cause of ischaemia in this context.

Q21. **Anatomy**

Answer: B. It is formed by the union of the maxillary vein and superficial temporal vein

Explanation: The retromandibular vein is formed by the confluence of the maxillary vein and the superficial temporal vein within the substance of the parotid gland. It descends posterior to the ramus of the mandible and divides into anterior and posterior branches. The posterior branch joins the posterior auricular vein to form the external jugular vein. The anterior branch contributes to the common facial vein, which drains into the internal jugular vein.

Q22. **Anatomy**

Answer: A. It drains directly into the subclavian vein

Explanation: The external jugular vein is formed by the union of the posterior auricular vein and the posterior division of the retromandibular vein near the angle of the mandible. It runs superficially along the sternocleidomastoid muscle and drains directly into the subclavian vein.

Q23. **Karapandzic flap**

Answer: A. Karapandzic flap

Explanation: The Karapandzic flap preserves the orbicularis oris muscle and its neurovascular supply, allowing for functional and aesthetic lower lip reconstruction. This technique maintains oral competence, sensation, and mobility, making it particularly suitable for defects involving up to 50% of the lip. In contrast, the Abbe flap is a cross-lip flap primarily used for central lip defects, while the Estlander flap is better suited for commissure reconstruction. The Abbe requires a second stage surgery, whereas the Estlander flap has the advantage of being a one-stage surgery, but the disadvantage of a resulting rounded commissure.

Q24. **Flap compromise**

Answer: B. Return to theatre for exploration

Explanation: Absent Doppler signals and signs of a compromised flap, such as coolness and pallor, indicate possible vascular compromise, necessitating urgent surgical exploration. Delaying intervention increases the risk of flap failure. Immediate return to the operating room allows identification and correction of issues such as thrombosis or anastomotic problems. Non-surgical measures, such as monitoring or imaging, are insufficient in the presence of such critical signs.

Q25. **Tracheostomy decannulation**

Answer: C. Ability to tolerate tracheostomy occlusion and clear secretions

Explanation: The most critical functional requirement for safe decannulation is the ability to protect the airway and clear secretions effectively. Without this, the patient is at risk of aspiration and respiratory compromise. Normal arterial blood gases are important but secondary to airway protection. The complete absence of respiratory secretions is not always feasible in patients with chronic conditions.

Q26. **Complications of tracheostomy**

Answer: C. Innominate artery

Explanation: The innominate (brachiocephalic) artery crosses anterior to the trachea at the sternal notch prior to dividing into right common carotid and subclavian arteries. High cuff pressures or oversized tracheostomy tubes may lead to erosion of the anterior tracheal wall resulting in tracheo-inominate artery fistula. This can present as massive haemorrhage which may have been preceded by haemoptysis or herald bleeds at the tracheostomy site.

Q27. **Options if no perforators found**

Answer: E. Use a fasciocutaneous paddle based on musculocutaneous perforators

Explanation: When no septocutaneous perforators are found during fibula free flap harvest, it is possible to include a fasciocutaneous paddle based on musculocutaneous perforators from the posterior crural septum. Abandoning the flap is unnecessary unless the vascular supply is entirely compromised. Intraoperative angiography may be helpful but is likely not to be practical in all settings.

Q28. **Options if poor collateral circulation**

Answer: B. Switch to an anterolateral thigh free flap

Explanation: Inadequate collateral circulation through the ulnar artery makes harvesting the radial artery for a free flap unsafe, as it could compromise hand perfusion. The anterolateral thigh (ALT) free flap is a suitable alternative, as it avoids the risk of vascular compromise in the hand. While a Doppler ultrasound may confirm the findings, it does not alter the management decision. Physiotherapy will not improve arterial supply, and switching to the right radial flap is not feasible due to the previous trauma.

Q29. **Options if inadequate bony reconstruction**

Answer: B. Augment the fibular graft with an iliac crest bone graft

Explanation: If the fibular free flap does not provide enough bone for the mandibular defect, it is common practice to augment it with an iliac crest bone graft for added bone stock. Bilateral fibular free flaps are not typically used due to the potential for increased morbidity. Switching to a scapular flap mid-procedure would complicate the surgery unnecessarily. Harvesting bone from the contralateral fibula is generally avoided to prevent bilateral leg weakness.

Q30. **Split-thickness skin grafts**

Answer: B. STSGs can tolerate up to four days of ischaemia before inosculation begins.

Explanation: STSGs consist of the epidermis and a portion of the dermis. Unlike FTSGs, STSGs rely entirely on the wound bed for revascularisation and lack their own blood supply. The graft initially survives via *imbibition*, absorbing oxygen and nutrients from the wound bed for up to four days. By around 48 hours, *inosculation* begins, establishing vascular connections between the graft and wound bed. The donor site of an STSG retains dermal appendages, including hair follicles, which facilitate reepithelialisation and allow the site to heal within two to three weeks, enabling reuse. Thin STSGs heal faster and have lower donor site morbidity but are less durable, making them unsuitable for mechanically demanding areas. Conversely, FTSGs provide a superior aesthetic match and durability, making them preferable for visible or high-stress areas. For STSG, absolute contraindications include wounds with an active infection, active bleeding, or known cancer, or wounds with exposed bone/tendon/nerve/blood vessel without appropriate vascular layer.

Q31. **Reconstruction of the eyebrow**

Answer: C. Pedicled scalp flap from the temporoparietal region

Explanation: In cases where the recipient bed is compromised, such as with significant scarring or thin skin, pedicled scalp flaps are preferred over free grafts due to their reliable blood supply, which increases the chances of graft survival. The pedicled flap also allows hair to grow in a more natural direction, minimising the risk of unnatural hair orientation. The postauricular temporoparietal region is a popular donor site because of its reliable vascular supply from the superficial temporal artery. Hair plug transplants or hair strip grafts are better suited for healthy, well-vascularised recipient beds and would be less likely to survive in a scarred area.

3 Oral Pathology and Bone Disease

QUESTIONS

Q1. A 14-year-old boy presents with fever and drooling. Over the past three days, he has developed bilateral preauricular swelling. He reports missing some vaccines in childhood, as his parents were concerned about potential side effects. Examination reveals tender, swollen parotid glands. Which of the following is a known complication of this disease?

A. Hepatitis
B. Gastroenteritis
C. Diverticulitis
D. Orchitis
E. Pneumonitis

Q2. A 5-year-old girl is brought to the clinic by her mother after receiving a letter from her child's playgroup regarding an outbreak of illness. The child has developed shallow, painful ulcers on her gingivae and tongue. On examination, you also observe vesicles on her hands and feet. Which virus is most likely responsible for this presentation?

A. Cytomegalovirus
B. Paramyxovirus
C. Epstein-Barr virus
D. Herpes simplex virus
E. Coxsackie A virus

Q3. A 72-year-old patient presents with a painful vesicular rash on the left side of their face, including lesions on the tip of the nose. The patient reports a burning sensation in the affected area. Which of the following is the best management option?

A. Prescribe oral antivirals and arrange routine follow-up
B. Refer urgently to an ophthalmologist
C. Prescribe topical steroids for symptomatic relief
D. Perform a bacterial swab and await results before starting treatment
E. Provide reassurance and monitor symptoms

Q4. A 25-year-old woman returns to the United Kingdom after a yearlong research placement in sub-Saharan Africa as part of her PhD. She has a history of systemic lupus erythematosus (SLE), well-controlled with long-term methotrexate and hydroxychloroquine. During a routine dental checkup, darkened areas are noted on her hard palate. Which of the following is the most likely explanation for this finding?

A. Early sign of Huntington's disease
B. Premalignant lesion

DOI: 10.1201/9781003609308-4

C. Adverse reaction to hydroxychloroquine
D. Adverse reaction to methotrexate
E. Early salivary gland tumour

Q5. A 27-year-old woman presents with a history of lethargy and joint pain. She reports noticing white lines on the inside of her cheek and a red rash under her eyes, which worsens significantly with sun exposure. What is the most likely diagnosis?
A. Acute drug reaction
B. Systemic lupus erythematosus (SLE)
C. Lead poisoning
D. Lichen planus
E. Measles infection

Q6. A midwife noticed a lesion inside the mouth of a newborn. The baby was born at term without complications six hours ago. The mother had normal antenatal screening, and no abnormalities were detected during pregnancy. The parents are distressed to see a thick, white, velvety lesion approximately 1 cm in size on the inside of the baby's left cheek, protruding into the oral cavity. What is the most likely diagnosis?
A. Frictional keratosis
B. Oral candidiasis
C. White sponge naevus
D. Congenital epulis
E. Proliferative verrucous leukoplakia

Q7. A 38-year-old patient with poorly controlled HIV presents with a painless white lesion on the lateral margin of the tongue. The lesion appears corrugated and cannot be scraped off. Which of the following conditions has the same causative agent as this oral lesion?
A. Nasopharyngeal carcinoma
B. Histoplasmosis
C. Cryptococcal meningitis
D. Kaposi sarcoma
E. Pneumocystis pneumonia

Q8. A 24-year-old woman presents with complaints of new-onset painful oral ulcers. Further history reveals itchy, sore, red eyes with blurred vision. She also reports recent genital ulcers after changing sexual partners and is awaiting results from a sexual health clinic. Family history includes Hashimoto's thyroiditis in her mother and asthma in her father. What is the most likely cause of her oral ulcers?
A. Hashimoto's thyroiditis
B. Chlamydia infection
C. Gonorrhoea infection
D. Stevens-Johnson syndrome (SJS)
E. Behçet's disease

Q9. A 27-year-old male sex worker presents for a dental checkup. On examination, you notice a punched-out, painless ulcer on the lateral surface of the tongue, which the patient reports has been present for two months without any change.

He denies weight loss, smoking, or any history of regular health checkups, including sexual health screening. Which of the following investigations is most likely to confirm the diagnosis?

A. Darkfield microscopy of the ulcer exudate
B. Polymerase chain reaction (PCR) for Epstein-Barr virus
C. Serum anti-nuclear antibody (ANA) test
D. Biopsy with histopathology
E. Treponemal serology

Q10. A 69-year-old male with a history of peripheral vascular disease, transient ischaemic attack, COPD, and sciatica presents with a right-sided headache that worsens with chewing. He reports a transient loss of vision in his right eye. Which of the following is the most specific test to confirm the causative disease?

A. ANCA
B. ESR
C. Temporal artery biopsy
D. CT head
E. Trial of carbamazepine

Q11. A 21-year-old refugee from Mali is referred with widespread white patches on the palate; these wipe off to leave an erythematous base. Despite treatment with nystatin and fluconazole, the condition has not improved. He reports a history of multiple severe chest infections. In addition to the aforementioned, which of the following findings are you most likely to observe on examination?

A. Yellow crusting lesions of the face
B. Oral hairy leukoplakia
C. Multiple small hyperpigmented lesions of the buccal mucosa
D. Bilateral enlarged parotid glands
E. Generalised gingival hypertrophy

Q12. A 30-year-old male is referred from his dentist with widespread alveolar bone loss, increased tooth mobility, oral ulceration, and a "strawberry" appearance to his gingivae. Which of the following is the most important investigation to include in your diagnostic workup?

A. Schirmer test
B. Anti-Ro antibodies
C. cANCA
D. ESR
E. Direct immunofluorescence

Q13. A 45-year-old man recently started on carbamazepine for trigeminal neuralgia presents with fever, malaise, and a widespread blistering rash involving his skin and oral mucosa. Examination reveals desquamation involving 8% of his total body surface area and erythema of the conjunctivae. Which of the following is the next best step in management?

A. Initiate oral antihistamines and observe for progression
B. Admit to intensive care unit for supportive care and fluid resuscitation
C. Administer broad-spectrum antibiotics immediately
D. Perform a skin biopsy to confirm the diagnosis
E. Start high-dose intravenous corticosteroids immediately

Q14. A 16-year-old male presents for evaluation of delayed eruption of permanent teeth. On examination, he demonstrates the ability to approximate his shoulders anteriorly. Radiographs reveal nine supernumerary teeth, delayed eruption of permanent teeth, and widened sutures of the skull. Which of the following additional findings would most strongly confirm the diagnosis?
A. Aortic root dilation
B. Hyperelastic skin and joint hypermobility
C. Complete or partial absence of clavicles
D. Hypoplasia of the zygomatic arches
E. Increased arm span-to-height ratio

Q15. A 24-year-old male presents with swelling in the anterior maxilla. A radiograph reveals a well-defined, unilocular radiolucency with flecks of calcification and evidence of root resorption in adjacent teeth. What is the most likely diagnosis?
A. Conventional ameloblastoma
B. Adenomatoid odontogenic tumour
C. Nasopalatine cyst
D. Simple bone cyst
E. Calcifying odontogenic cyst

Q16. A 5-year-old boy presents with a mixed radiopacity lesion in the anterior mandible. A histology report from the lesion reveals the presence of enamel and dentine. Which of the following is the most likely diagnosis?
A. Ameloblastoma
B. Ameloblastic fibroma
C. Ameloblastic fibro-odontoma
D. Residual cyst
E. Stafne's bone cavity

Q17. A 33-year-old male presents with significant swelling in the left lower quadrant (LLQ) of the mandible. Examination reveals a smooth, hard buccal sulcus swelling with a central soft, compressible area less than 1 cm in diameter. No "eggshell cracking" is noted. An orthopantogram (OPG) shows a multilocular radiolucency in the body of the mandible with radiopaque septa. Which of the following features would most strongly support the correct diagnosis?
A. Histological presence of stellate and spindle cells within an extracellular matrix
B. Presence of giant cells in a fibrovascular stroma on biopsy
C. Detection of PTCH1 gene mutation on genetic testing
D. Symmetrical, bilateral lesions involving the mandible and maxilla
E. Histological identification of palisading columnar basal cells with reverse nuclear polarity

Q18. A 13-year-old presents with a sore throat, fever, and bilateral cervical lymphadenopathy. Examination reveals enlarged tonsils with a grey-white exudate. A rapid strep test is negative. What is the most likely causative pathogen?
A. Adenovirus
B. Streptococcus pyogenes
C. Corynebacterium diphtheriae
D. Epstein-Barr virus
E. Fusobacterium necrophorum

Q19. A 33-year-old female presents with painful white plaques on the tongue and buccal mucosa that can be scraped off, revealing erythematous mucosa. She is in her first trimester. Which of the following is the most appropriate treatment option?

A. Itraconazole
B. Fluconazole
C. Amphotericin B
D. Nystatin
E. Chlorhexidine mouthwash

Q20. A 30-year-old patient presents with painless swelling in the anterior mandible. Imaging reveals a multilocular radiolucent lesion. Biopsy confirms central giant cell granuloma. What is the most appropriate initial management?

A. Calcitonin therapy
B. Denosumab therapy
C. Intralesional corticosteroid injection
D. Enucleation and curettage
E. Resection with reconstruction

Q21. A 15-year-old male presents with painless bilateral mandibular expansion and worsening malocclusion. Imaging reveals a mixed radiopacity lesion. Biopsy shows fibrocellular stroma with irregular woven bone. What is the most likely diagnosis?

A. Fibrous dysplasia
B. Cherubism
C. Ossifying fibroma
D. Central giant cell granuloma
E. Paget's disease

Q22. A 13-year-old male presents with multiple painful ulcers on the tongue and buccal mucosa. He also has fever and cervical lymphadenopathy. Which of the following is the most likely cause?

A. Epstein-Barr virus (EBV)
B. Mycoplasma pneumoniae
C. Herpes simplex virus (HSV)
D. Coxsackievirus
E. Candida albicans

Q23. A 68-year-old male with hypertension reports dry mouth and difficulty swallowing. Which of the following is most likely causing his symptoms?

A. Atenolol
B. Ramipril
C. Amlodipine
D. Hydrochlorothiazide
E. Losartan

Q24. A 55-year-old female is referred due to painful oral erosions. She recently was recently started on a new disease modifying anti-rheumatic drug (DMARD). Which of the following drugs is most likely responsible?

A. Methotrexate
B. Hydroxychloroquine
C. Prednisolone

D. Etanercept
E. Sulfasalazine

Q25. A 26-year-old female with advanced HIV presents with a painful ulcer on the hard palate. Biopsy shows fungal hyphae invading the tissue. What is the most likely organism, and what systemic complication is the patient most at risk for?
A. Candida albicans; candidemia
B. Aspergillus fumigatus; pulmonary aspergillosis
C. Cryptococcus neoformans; meningitis
D. Mucor species; rhinocerebral mucormycosis
E. Histoplasma capsulatum; disseminated histoplasmosis

Q26. A 62-year-old male with tense bullae and erythematous areas on the gingivae undergoes biopsy. Histology shows subepithelial clefting and linear IgG deposition at the basement membrane. Which of the following is the most likely diagnosis?
A. Pemphigus vulgaris
B. Bullous pemphigoid
C. Erythema multiforme
D. Herpes simplex gingivostomatitis
E. Mucous membrane pemphigoid

Q27. A 50-year-old male presents with flaccid bullae and erosions on the oral mucosa. Biopsy shows acantholysis and suprabasal clefting. Immunofluorescence reveals IgG deposition in a fishnet pattern. What additional diagnostic test is most important to guide systemic management?
A. ANA and ENA panel
B. Serum anti-BP180 and anti-BP230
C. Serum anti-desmoglein antibody testing
D. Biopsy from unaffected mucosa
E. Viral serology for HSV

Q28. A 34-year-old male presents with a painless, white, verrucous lesion on the buccal mucosa. Biopsy reveals hyperkeratosis and acanthosis but no dysplasia. He reports a history of betel nut chewing. What is the best management strategy for this lesion?
A. Observation and regular follow-up
B. Topical corticosteroids
C. Surgical excision
D. Antifungal therapy
E. Cryotherapy

Q29. A 70-year-old female presents with jaw claudication, scalp tenderness, and new-onset headache. ESR is elevated at 78 mm/hr. What is the most important next step in management?
A. Temporal artery biopsy
B. Start high-dose corticosteroids
C. CT angiogram
D. Low-dose aspirin therapy
E. MRI of the head

Q30. A 45-year-old female presents with decreased taste sensation on the anterior two-thirds of her tongue and ipsilateral dry eyes. Damage to which of the following nerves is most likely responsible for her symptoms?

A. Lingual nerve
B. Facial nerve at the geniculate ganglion
C. Hypoglossal nerve
D. Glossopharyngeal nerve
E. Chorda tympani

Q31. A 67-year-old male presents with sharp, stabbing pain in the right lower jaw and chin, triggered by brushing his teeth and talking. Neurological examination is normal. MRI reveals vascular compression of the right trigeminal nerve root by the superior cerebellar artery. Which of the following best explains the pathophysiology of his condition?

A. Ectopic generation of action potentials due to demyelination
B. Increased excitability of nociceptive C fibres
C. Chronic ischaemia of the trigeminal ganglion
D. Inflammatory cytokine release around the nerve root
E. Synaptic reorganisation in the central trigeminal nuclei

Q32. A 38-year-old male presents with severe unilateral orbital and temporal pain lasting for 30 minutes, accompanied by ipsilateral lacrimation and nasal congestion. Symptoms occur daily for several weeks. Which of the following is the most appropriate medication to prevent recurrence of symptoms?

A. Verapamil
B. Sumatriptan
C. Amitriptyline
D. Prednisolone
E. Carbamazepine

Q33. A 35-year-old male presents with a progressively enlarging swelling of the right mandible, associated with increasing mobility of the lower right molars and premolars. Despite a course of antibiotics, there has been no improvement. Radiographs reveal a large unilocular lesion with destruction of the tooth roots and a "sunburst" appearance. Biopsy is performed.

Which of the following is **true** regarding the likely diagnosis?

A. Histology confirms heavy abundance of osteoid.
B. Histology confirms cells arranged in a follicular pattern within a connective tissue stroma with central cells resembling the stellate reticulum.
C. This lesion has a higher risk of metastasis when present in the jaws compared to other primary locations.
D. Marginal resection is sufficient for curative management.
E. The lesion typically lacks any soft tissue involvement.

ANSWERS AND EXPLANATIONS

Q1. **Mumps**

Answer: D. Orchitis

Explanation: This presentation is consistent with mumps, a viral infection characterised by parotitis, often occurring in unvaccinated individuals. Complications of mumps include orchitis (inflammation of the testes, particularly in postpubertal males), meningitis, oophoritis, pancreatitis, and hearing loss. The other listed conditions are not typically associated with mumps.

Q2. **Hand foot and mouth disease**

Answer: E. Coxsackie A virus

Explanation: This child has hand, foot, and mouth disease (HFMD), which is caused by Coxsackie A virus, most commonly Coxsackie A16. HFMD typically presents with painful oral ulcers and vesicular lesions on the hands, feet, and sometimes the buttocks.

Q3. **Herpes zoster**

Answer: B. Refer urgently to an ophthalmologist

Explanation: The presence of vesicles on the tip of the nose (Hutchinson's sign) in the context of shingles (herpes zoster) is a red flag for potential ophthalmic involvement, as it indicates nasociliary nerve involvement. This increases the risk of herpes zoster ophthalmicus, which can lead to corneal damage and blindness if untreated. Oral antivirals are part of the treatment and should be prescribed within 72 hours of onset of vesicles, but urgent ophthalmology referral is crucial due to the risk of eye involvement. Oral steroids were previously thought to be of benefit in minimising risk of postherpetic neuralgia. However, a recent Cochrane review (6) found uncertainty about the effects. As a result, NICE could not find sufficient evidence to support a recommendation for oral corticosteroids for the treatment of acute pain in people with shingles, "so the recommendation to consider offering corticosteroids based on clinical judgment is pragmatic".

Q4. **Drug-induced oral pigmentation**

Answer: C. Adverse reaction to hydroxychloroquine

Explanation: In this case, the hyperpigmented lesions on the hard palate are most likely a side effect of hydroxychloroquine, a drug commonly used in the management of SLE. Oral hyperpigmentation is a well-documented adverse effect of long-term antimalarial medications. Premalignant lesions should be considered in patients on immunosuppressants like methotrexate; however, in this case, the hyperpigmentation is a known drug side effect. Methotrexate can cause oral ulceration or mucositis but is not associated with hyperpigmentation.

Q5. **Systemic lupus erythematosus**

Answer: B. Systemic lupus erythematosus (SLE)

Explanation: SLE is an autoimmune disorder that presents with a wide range of nonspecific symptoms. Key features in this case include the following:

- Malar rash: A classic butterfly-shaped rash over the cheeks and nose, sparing the nasolabial folds, and often exacerbated by sunlight.
- White lines on the buccal mucosa: These could be secondary to mucosal involvement, occasionally seen in SLE.

Other options explained:

- A. Acute drug reaction: Typically associated with urticarial or maculopapular rashes but not specific for SLE features like the malar rash.
- C. Lead poisoning: Presents with a bluish-grey "Burton's line" on the gingivae, not white lines on the buccal mucosa or a malar rash.
- D. Lichen planus: Although a far more common cause of white lesions on the buccal mucosa, lacks the systemic symptoms and sun-exacerbated rash of SLE.
- E. Measles infection: Typically causes Koplik spots on the buccal mucosa, fever, and a diffuse maculopapular rash—not the malar rash seen here.

Q6. **White sponge naevus**

Answer: C. White sponge naevus

Explanation: White sponge naevus is caused by a genetic mutation resulting in abnormal keratinisation of the oral mucosa. It typically presents as thick, velvety, sponge-like plaques, often from birth or early childhood. Lesions may be bilateral and are not associated with systemic abnormalities or malignancy.

- A. Frictional keratosis: Caused by chronic irritation (e.g., biting or rubbing), uncommon in newborns.
- B. Oral candidiasis: Presents with white plaques that scrape off, revealing erythematous mucosa. This lesion does not fit the description of a velvety, thick, and non-removable plaque.
- D. Congenital epulis: Presents as a pedunculated, reddish-pink mass on the alveolar ridge, not as a white velvety lesion.
- E. Proliferative verrucous leukoplakia: A progressive and premalignant condition that develops over time, typically in adults.

Q7. **Epstein-Barr virus**

Answer: A. Nasopharyngeal carcinoma

Explanation: The patient's presentation is consistent with OHL, a condition caused by EBV, commonly seen in immunosuppressed individuals such as those with HIV/AIDS. OHL presents as a white, corrugated lesion on the lateral tongue that cannot be scraped off. It is not premalignant but is a marker of advanced immunosuppression.

A. Nasopharyngeal carcinoma: This malignancy is also associated with EBV, particularly in endemic regions. Both nasopharyngeal carcinoma and OHL share the same viral aetiology.

Other options:

- B. Histoplasmosis: Caused by Histoplasma capsulatum, a fungal infection seen in immunocompromised patients but unrelated to EBV.
- C. Cryptococcal meningitis: Caused by Cryptococcus neoformans, a fungal infection affecting the central nervous system in advanced HIV, not associated with EBV.
- D. Kaposi sarcoma: Caused by Kaposi sarcoma-associated herpesvirus (HHV-8), presenting as vascular lesions, not related to EBV.
- E. Pneumocystis pneumonia: Caused by Pneumocystis jirovecii, a fungal infection in the lungs, unrelated to EBV.

Q8. **Behçet's disease**

Answer: E. Behçet's disease

Explanation: This patient's symptoms of recurrent oral ulcers, genital ulcers, and ocular inflammation (likely uveitis) point towards a diagnosis of Behçet's disease, an autoinflammatory vasculitis. Behçet's disease is most common in young adults and has a higher prevalence in Middle Eastern and Mediterranean populations, particularly Turkey, though it can occur worldwide. Management with a multidisciplinary approach is essential, often involving steroids (topical, oral, or IV) for mucocutaneous disease, colchicine for inflammation, and escalation to TNF inhibitors (e.g., infliximab) for refractory cases. Prognosis is variable, with relapsing and remitting patterns; however, significant CNS or vascular involvement carries higher morbidity.

Differential Diagnoses:

- A. Hashimoto's thyroiditis: Autoimmune thyroiditis does not explain the triad of symptoms.
- B. Chlamydia infection: May cause genital ulcers but not oral ulcers involvement.
- C. Gonorrhoea infection: Can cause genital inflammation but does not explain the oral findings.
- D. SJS: Causes mucocutaneous lesions but is usually linked to drug reactions or infections and involves widespread skin detachment.

Q9. **Syphilis**

Answer: E. Treponemal serology

Explanation: The most likely diagnosis is primary syphilis, presenting with a painless chancre. Treponemal serology is a highly sensitive and specific test to confirm the diagnosis. Darkfield microscopy, while useful in the diagnosis of syphilis, is less commonly employed in modern practice due to technical challenges. PCR for EBV and ANA testing are unrelated to this presentation, and biopsy with histopathology may be useful to exclude malignancy, but the stem is strongly suggestive of syphilis as the cause.

Q10. **Temporal arteritis**

Answer: C. Temporal artery biopsy

Explanation: This patient's symptoms are highly suggestive of temporal arteritis (giant cell arteritis), which commonly presents with headache, jaw claudication, and visual disturbances due to inflammation of the temporal arteries. While ESR is a sensitive test often elevated in temporal arteritis, it is not specific. Temporal artery biopsy is the most specific test, confirming the diagnosis with histological evidence of inflammation and giant cells. ANCA testing is more relevant for small vessel vasculitis, while carbamazepine trials are for trigeminal neuralgia. CT head is useful to investigate haemorrhagic and ischaemic stroke but not diagnostic for temporal arteritis.

Q11. **HIV**

Answer: B. Oral hairy leukoplakia

Explanation: The patient's symptoms strongly suggest immunosuppression, necessitating a HIV test. OHL is a classic finding in immunocompromised individuals and is caused by EBV reactivation. Yellow crusting lesions (e.g., impetigo) are unrelated to this context, and gingival hypertrophy is more typical of certain medications (e.g., phenytoin, cyclosporine) or leukaemia's. Hyperpigmented lesions suggest conditions like Addison's disease, and bilateral parotid gland enlargement may indicate Sjögren's syndrome or sarcoidosis, which are less consistent with this presentation.

Q12. **Granulomatosis with polyangiitis**

Answer: C. cANCA

Explanation: This presentation is characteristic of GPA, which often involves oral manifestations such as a "strawberry" gingiva, ulceration, and alveolar bone loss. Classically, it causes pathology of the lungs, kidneys, nose and sinuses. cANCA testing (specifically for anti-proteinase three antibodies) is highly sensitive and specific for diagnosing GPA. Schirmer testing and anti-Ro antibodies are associated with Sjögren's syndrome, which does not explain the bone loss or gingival appearance. ESR is nonspecific, and direct immunofluorescence is more relevant for suspected vesiculobullous diseases such as pemphigus or pemphigoid.

Q13. **Stevens-Johnson syndrome**

Answer: B. Admit to an intensive care unit for supportive care and fluid resuscitation

Explanation: This presentation is consistent with SJS, a severe mucocutaneous reaction often triggered by drugs including anti-epileptics (e.g. carbamazepine, lamotrigine, and phenytoin), anti-gout medications (e.g. allopurinol), antibiotics (e.g. sulfamethoxazole, minocycline, and β-lactam antibiotics) and non-steroidal anti-inflammatory drugs. Initial management involves supportive care in a burns or intensive care unit, including fluid resuscitation and monitoring for complications. IV corticosteroids and IVIG may form part of the treatment protocol. Antibiotics and antifungals may be required for superinfection. Treatment should not be delayed for a biopsy.

Q14. **Cleidocranial dysplasia**

Answer: C. Complete or partial absence of clavicles

Explanation: This presentation is consistent with cleidocranial dysplasia, a genetic disorder caused by mutations in the RUNX2 gene, affecting bone and dental development. The ability to approximate the shoulders anteriorly is due to hypoplasia or absence of the clavicles. Other classic features include supernumerary teeth, delayed eruption, hypertelorism, a retruded maxilla, and skull abnormalities (e.g., widened sutures, persistent fontanelles).

- A. Aortic root dilation: Seen in Marfan syndrome, not associated with cleidocranial dysplasia.
- B. Hyperelastic skin and joint hypermobility: A feature of Ehlers-Danlos syndrome.
- D. Hypoplasia of the zygomatic arches: Seen in Treacher Collins syndrome, not cleidocranial dysplasia.
- E. Increased arm span-to-height ratio: Typical of Marfan syndrome but not relevant here.

Q15. **Calcifying odontogenic cyst**

Answer: E. Calcifying odontogenic cyst

Explanation: The findings are consistent with a COC, also known as Gorlin's cyst. COCs typically occur in the anterior maxilla and appear as well-circumscribed, unilocular radiolucencies with scattered calcifications that can vary in size based on the lesion's maturity. They may resorb or displace adjacent teeth. Histologically, they are characterised by "ghost cells," which are eosinophilic, enlarged cells without nuclei. Management involves enucleation.

Q16. **Ameloblastic fibro-odontoma**

Answer: C. Ameloblastic fibro-odontoma

Explanation: Ameloblastic fibro-odontoma is a rare odontogenic tumour primarily seen in children. It resembles ameloblastic fibromas but is distinguished by the presence of enamel or dentine within the lesion, visible histologically and radiographically as radiopacities. These radiopacities can appear as a solid mass or multiple discrete areas and are often associated with an unerupted tooth.

Q17. **Odontogenic myxoma**

Answer: A. Histological presence of stellate and spindle cells within a myxoid stroma

Explanation: The clinical and radiographic findings are consistent with odontogenic myxoma, a rare odontogenic tumour characterised histologically by stellate and spindle cells embedded in a myxoid or mucoid extracellular matrix. The lesion commonly occurs in young adults and presents radiographically as a multilocular radiolucency with a "tennis racquet" pattern due to perpendicular radiopaque septa.

- B. Presence of giant cells in a fibrovascular stroma: Suggestive of a central giant cell granuloma.
- C. Detection of PTCH1 gene mutation: Associated with Gorlin-Goltz syndrome, which presents with multiple odontogenic keratocysts and basal cell carcinomas.
- D. Symmetrical, bilateral lesions involving the mandible and maxilla: Typical of cherubism, not odontogenic myxoma.
- E. Histological identification of palisading columnar basal cells with reverse nuclear polarity: Indicative of ameloblastoma, not odontogenic myxoma.

Q18. **Epstein-Barr virus**

Answer: D. Epstein-Barr virus

Explanation: EBV causes infectious mononucleosis, characterised by pharyngitis, fever, and cervical lymphadenopathy. The negative strep test and presence of exudates point to EBV. Streptococcus pyogenes would test positive on a rapid strep test. Corynebacterium diphtheriae causes pseudomembranous pharyngitis but is rare due to vaccination. Adenovirus causes viral pharyngitis but classically lacks exudates (although that is not always the case). Fusobacterium necrophorum is a bacterium that is associated with tonsillitis, peritonsillar abscesses, and Lemierre's syndrome (involving jugular vein thrombophlebitis).

Q19. **Oral candidiasis**

Answer: D. Nystatin

Explanation: Oral candidiasis in pregnancy is best treated with topical antifungals such as nystatin, as systemic absorption from the gastrointestinal tract is negligible. However, the manufacturer advises its use in pregnancy only if the potential benefits outweigh the possible risks, as its effects on fetal development are not well studied. Fluconazole, in contrast, is contraindicated due to its teratogenic potential, and women should observe a washout period of approximately one week after discontinuation before becoming pregnant. Itraconazole and amphotericin B are generally reserved for refractory or systemic infections. Chlorhexidine mouthwash may provide symptomatic relief but is not a definitive treatment for oral candidiasis.

Q20. **Central giant cell granuloma**

Answer: D. Enucleation and curettage

Explanation: Central giant cell granuloma is a benign but occasionally aggressive lesion. The initial treatment is surgical enucleation and curettage. Resection is reserved for extensive, destructive lesions. Medical therapies including corticosteroids, calcitonin injection, and denosumab have been trialled with varying success.

Q21. **Fibrous dysplasia**

Answer: A. Fibrous dysplasia

Explanation: Fibrous dysplasia presents with gradual, painless expansion of affected bones, commonly involving the mandible. The ground glass or peau d'orange radiographic appearance and histology of fibrocellular stroma with woven bone are diagnostic. Cherubism (B) causes bilateral mandibular expansion but is typically associated with younger children and familial history. Ossifying fibroma (C) presents as a well-circumscribed lesion with a mixed radiolucent and radiopaque appearance. Central giant cell granuloma (D) is often more aggressive with cortical perforation, and Paget's disease (E) typically occurs in older adults with mixed radiographic changes.

Q22. **Herpes simplex virus**

Answer: C. Herpes simplex virus (HSV)

Explanation: Primary herpetic gingivostomatitis, caused by HSV, presents with widespread painful oral ulcers, fever, and lymphadenopathy.

Q23. **Xerostomia**

Answer: D. Hydrochlorothiazide

Explanation: Hydrochlorothiazide, a thiazide diuretic, is commonly associated with xerostomia due to its dehydrating effect, which reduces salivary gland output.

Q24. **Oral mucositis**

Answer: A. Methotrexate

Explanation: Methotrexate is a folate antagonist commonly used as a DMARD, and it is well known for causing oral mucositis and ulceration, especially at higher doses or in patients with inadequate folate supplementation. This side effect results from methotrexate's inhibition of rapidly dividing epithelial cells in the oral mucosa. In contrast, hydroxychloroquine and sulfasalazine are less likely to cause mucositis, while corticosteroids like prednisolone are more often associated with oral candidiasis due to immunosuppression. Etanercept, a TNF-α inhibitor, can cause immunosuppression

Q25. **Mucormycosis**

Answer: D. Mucor species; rhinocerebral mucormycosis

Explanation: Mucormycosis often affects immunosuppressed individuals, causing characteristic tissue necrosis and rapid progression to rhinocerebral or disseminated disease. Mucormycetes species that may opportunistically result in mucormycosis include Rhizopus oryzae and Rhizopus delemar.

Q26. **Mucous membrane pemphigoid**

Answer: E. Mucous membrane pemphigoid

Explanation: Mucous membrane pemphigoid presents with subepithelial clefting and linear IgG deposition at the basement membrane targeting BP 180 and 230.

Q27. **Pemphigus vulgaris**

Answer: C. Serum anti-desmoglein antibody testing

Explanation: Pemphigus vulgaris is associated with autoantibodies against desmoglein. Measuring these antibodies can help confirm the diagnosis and monitor disease activity.

Q28. **Proliferative verrucous leukoplakia**

Answer: C. Surgical excision

Explanation: Verrucous hyperplasia is a part of the developmental spectrum of proliferative verrucous leukoplakia (PVL), a potentially malignant lesion. Surgical excision with adequate margins is the definitive treatment.

Q29. **Giant cell arteritis**

Answer: B. Start high-dose corticosteroids

Explanation: The presentation is consistent with giant cell arteritis. Immediate high-dose corticosteroids should be started to prevent vision loss, even before biopsy confirmation.

Q30. **Facial nerve anatomy**

Answer: B. Facial nerve at the geniculate ganglion

Explanation: The facial nerve at the geniculate ganglion gives rise to the chorda tympani, which supplies taste sensation to the anterior two-thirds of the tongue and parasympathetic fibres to the submandibular and sublingual glands. Damage here can also affect the greater petrosal nerve, leading to dry eyes.

Q31. **Trigeminal neuralgia**

Answer: A. Ectopic generation of action potentials due to demyelination

Explanation: There is growing evidence that trigeminal neuralgia usually caused by demyelination of the trigeminal sensory fibres within the nerve root or brainstem. This is often attributed to compression by the superior cerebellar artery, leading to focal demyelination. Ephaptic transmission occurs when demyelinated axons in the trigeminal nerve generate ectopic impulses that can be transferred to nearby pain fibres. This happens when action potentials jump from one fibre to another, altering the excitability of neighbouring neurons. This results in the characteristic paroxysmal stabbing pain. Treatments like carbamazepine target this hyperexcitability, while microvascular decompression addresses the underlying vascular compression in refractory cases.

Q32. **Cluster headaches**

Answer: A. Verapamil

Explanation: Verapamil is the first-line prophylactic treatment for cluster headaches, as it reduces the frequency and severity of attacks. Sumatriptan (B) is used for acute treatment, not prophylaxis.

Q33. **Osteosarcoma**

Answer: A. Histology confirms heavy abundance of osteoid.

Explanation: Osteosarcoma of the mandible is a rare malignant bone tumour characterised by the production of osteoid matrix, which is a diagnostic hallmark confirmed on histology. The "sunburst" radiographic appearance is typical but not exclusive to osteosarcoma. Marginal resection is insufficient; wide surgical resection with adjuvant chemotherapy is required due to its aggressive nature and risk of recurrence (7). Compared to primary lesions of long bones, mandibular osteosarcomas are significantly smaller tumours and are far less likely to metastasise. Option B is describing histological features of ameloblastoma.

4 Cutaneous

QUESTIONS

Q1. A 27-year-old fit and well female presents with a slow-growing, firm lesion in the right eyebrow region, measuring approximately 4 cm by 2 cm. The lump is mobile, with erythematous overlying skin and normal hair growth. There is no visible punctum. Imaging confirms no bony involvement. Fine needle cytology reveals cells resembling hair matrix and eosinophilic cells without nuclei. What is the most appropriate next step in management?
A. Excisional biopsy via an upper blepharoplasty incision
B. Core biopsy to confirm the diagnosis
C. Incisional biopsy to reduce lesion size
D. Observation with follow-up imaging
E. Wide local excision with 5 mm margins

Q2. A 12-year-old female presents with a red, soft, non-pulsatile lesion in the right infraorbital region, first noticed around 1 year of age. The lesion has continued to grow and is now approaching the lower eyelid. The patient has been on oral atenolol for the past year, with minimal reduction in lesion size. Her parents are concerned due to the lesion's proximity to the eye. What is the most appropriate next step in management?
A. Intralesional betamethasone
B. Observation with annual follow-up
C. Oral propranolol
D. Surgical excision and laser therapy
E. Systemic corticosteroids

Q3. A 21-year-old female presents for review following an upper lip injury from a hockey stick 12 months ago. The laceration was closed primarily at the time of injury but became infected, requiring antibiotics two weeks post-injury. She is unhappy with the scar's appearance due to its colour and texture. On examination, the left upper lip shows eversion and a distorted margin. What is the most appropriate next step in management?
A. Chemical peel
B. Dermabrasion
C. Laser therapy
D. Skin bleaching agents
E. Z-plasty

Q4. A 67-year-old male presents with a 1.4 cm basal cell carcinoma (BCC) near the alar rim of the nose. Following excision, a full-thickness defect is anticipated. What is the most appropriate method for reconstructing this defect?

DOI: 10.1201/9781003609308-5

A. Split-thickness skin graft from the supraclavicular region
B. Preauricular full-thickness skin graft
C. Composite graft from the auricular helix
D. Bilobed flap
E. Nasolabial flap

Q5. A 73-year-old male undergoes Moh's resection for a basal cell carcinoma of the upper eyelid. The defect measures less than 25% of the horizontal dimension of the lid; the lid margin is not involved; the tarsal plate has been kept intact. Which of the following is the best management option?
A. Direct closure of the defect
B. Lateral cantholysis with medial transposition of the upper lid
C. Lid switch procedure from the lower eyelid
D. Cutler-Beard flap
E. Nasolabial flap with mucosal graft

Q6. A 40-year-old gardener presents with a red, erythematous rash on the right cheek accompanied by fever and regional lymphadenopathy. There is a central area of ulceration. What is the most likely causative pathogen?
A. Borrelia burgdorferi
B. Bacillus anthracis
C. Sporothrix schenckii
D. Streptococcus pyogenes
E. Rickettsia rickettsii

Q7. A 5-year-old child presents with multiple small, shiny, dome-shaped papules with a central umbilicated area. They originated on the trunk and have now spread to the neck and face. There are no systemic symptoms. What is the most likely causative pathogen?
A. Human papillomavirus
B. Poxvirus
C. Herpes simplex virus
D. Varicella-zoster virus
E. Coxsackievirus

Q8. A 70-year-old patient presents with a rapidly growing, painless, firm, violaceous nodule on the face. Histopathology is still awaited. Which virus is most commonly associated with this malignancy?
A. Epstein-Barr virus
B. Human herpesvirus 8
C. Merkel cell polyomavirus
D. Human papillomavirus
E. Cytomegalovirus

Q9. A 68-year-old patient presents with a rapidly growing, painless, violaceous nodule on the forehead. A biopsy confirms malignancy and neuroendocrine markers. What is the most appropriate next management?
A. Wide local excision with 1 cm margins

B. Wide local excision with 2 cm margins, sentinel lymph node biopsy and adjuvant radiotherapy
C. Primary radiotherapy alone to the lesion
D. Systemic chemotherapy with cisplatin-based regimens
E. Immunotherapy with avelumab

Q10. A 73-year-old male with atrial fibrillation is currently on rivaroxaban. He presents with a 2 cm ulcerated, biopsy-proven squamous cell carcinoma (SCC) on the left pinna. Which of the following is the most appropriate management option for this patient?
A. Surgical excision with a 5 mm margin
B. Surgical excision with a 6 mm margin
C. Surgical excision with a 4 mm margin and adjuvant radiotherapy
D. Systemic treatment with cemiplimab
E. Mohs surgery

Q11. A 65-year-old male presents with a 1.5 cm well-defined, biopsy-proven cutaneous squamous cell carcinoma (SCC) on his left cheek. There is no evidence of perineural invasion, and it appears well differentiated. What is the most appropriate management for this patient?
A. Curettage and cautery
B. Surgical excision with a 2 mm margin
C. Surgical excision with a 4 mm margin
D. Surgical excision with a 6 mm margin
E. Radiotherapy

Q12. A patient is referred from dermatology with multiple basal cell carcinomas (BCCs). Investigations have also revealed palmar pitting and a multiloculated radiolucency at the left mandibular angle. Which of the following is most likely?
A. Sweet's syndrome
B. Tuberous sclerosis
C. Nevoid basal cell carcinoma syndrome
D. Cowden syndrome
E. Gardner syndrome

Q13. A 62-year-old female presents with a biopsy-proven morpheic basal cell carcinoma (BCC) on the left dorsum of the nose. She has a history of a previous BCC removal from the dorsal surface of the nose four years ago. What is the most appropriate management for this lesion?
A. Excision with a 3 mm margin
B. Excision with a 5 mm margin
C. Excision with a 10 mm margin
D. Mohs micrographic surgery
E. Curettage and cautery

Q14. A 72-year-old patient presents with a pigmented lesion on the right cheek that is clinically suspicious for melanoma. There is no history of previous excision or biopsy of the lesion. What is the most appropriate initial management for this patient?

A. Observation with follow-up in 3 months
B. Excision with a 2 mm margin
C. Excision with a 5 mm margin
D. Incisional biopsy from the most abnormal area
E. Wide local excision with reconstruction

Q15. A 62-year-old patient with a history of rheumatoid arthritis treated with methotrexate and biologic therapy has been diagnosed with a biopsy-proven melanoma on their left forearm. The lesion measures 2.5 mm in Breslow thickness. What is the most appropriate management for this patient?
A. Wide local excision with a 1 cm margin
B. Wide local excision with a 1–2 cm margin
C. Wide local excision with a 2–3 cm margin
D. Observation with regular dermatology follow-up
E. Mohs micrographic surgery

Q16. A 62-year-old male presents with a confirmed metastatic melanoma in the left cervical lymph nodes after excision of a 2.5 mm thick melanoma on the cheek. What is the most appropriate management of the nodal disease?
A. Adjuvant radiotherapy
B. Immunotherapy with checkpoint inhibitors
C. Therapeutic lymphadenectomy of the cervical lymph nodes
D. Sentinel lymph node biopsy
E. Chemotherapy

Q17. A 32-year-old male presents with multiple painful vesicles on the left forehead, accompanied by ipsilateral conjunctival injection and photophobia. He has a history of poorly controlled diabetes. What is the most appropriate next step in management?
A. Oral valacyclovir and urgent ophthalmology referral
B. Topical acyclovir and observation
C. Empirical antibiotics for secondary infection
D. Surgical debridement of necrotic tissue
E. Oral acyclovir and admission for IV antibiotics

Q18. A 42-year-old male presents with a slow-growing, well-circumscribed, dome-shaped lesion on the forehead. The lesion is firm, non-tender, and has a central keratin plug. Biopsy reveals keratin-filled cystic spaces lined by squamous epithelium with no atypia. What is the most appropriate management?
A. Observation and follow-up
B. Cryotherapy
C. Curettage and cautery
D. Wide local excision with histopathology
E. Radiotherapy

Q19. A 68-year-old male with a history of extensive sun exposure presents with a scaly, erythematous patch on his scalp that does not heal. Biopsy confirms actinic keratosis with moderate dysplasia. What is the most appropriate first-line treatment?
A. Observation with regular follow-up
B. Topical 5-fluorouracil

C. Mohs micrographic surgery
D. Wide local excision with 4 mm margins
E. Sentinel lymph node biopsy

Q20. A 74-year-old male presents with a 4.5 cm ulcerated lesion on the posterior scalp. Biopsy confirms squamous cell carcinoma with moderate differentiation. Imaging reveals no evidence of distant metastases, but MRI shows extensive perineural invasion. Which treatment option is most appropriate for optimal local control?

A. Wide local excision with 1 cm margins
B. Mohs micrographic surgery
C. Wide local excision with adjuvant radiotherapy
D. Sentinel lymph node biopsy
E. Radiotherapy alone

Q21. A 72-year-old patient with a 3 cm squamous cell carcinoma (SCC) of the scalp is scheduled for resection and reconstruction with a large local flap. The patient is on rivaroxaban for atrial fibrillation, with an eGFR of 50 mL/min. What is the most appropriate perioperative management of dabigatran in this case?

A. Continue rivaroxaban without interruption.
B. Stop rivaroxaban one day before surgery and restart six hours postoperatively.
C. Stop rivaroxaban two days before surgery and restart when adequate haemostasis is achieved immediately postoperatively.
D. Stop rivaroxaban 3 days before surgery and 24–48 hours postoperatively.
E. Administer prothrombin complex concentrate (PCC) preoperatively to reverse rivaroxaban and restart 24 hours postoperatively.

Q22. A 63-year-old female patient presents with significant chronic infection and wound breakdown at the donor site following reconstruction of an oral squamous cell carcinoma (OSCC) with a fibula free flap. After surgical debridement, a vacuum-assisted closure (VAC) dressing is applied to the donor site. Which of the following statements is true regarding the use of vacuum-assisted closure (VAC) therapy in this case?

A. Negative-pressure wound therapy (NPWT) is contraindicated for infected wounds and should be avoided.
B. The optimal pressure for wound healing using NPWT is approximately 85 mmHg with an alternating pressure cycle of 5 minutes suction followed by 2 minutes off.
C. VAC therapy promotes wound healing primarily by increasing the extracellular fluid content in the wound.
D. NPWT should be set to continuous suction to facilitate the healing of the donor site.
E. VAC therapy should not be used on directly exposed bone or tendons, as it may cause damage to these structures.

ANSWERS AND EXPLANATIONS

Q1. **Benign tumour of eyebrow**

Answer: A. Excisional biopsy via an upper blepharoplasty incision

Explanation: The clinical and cytological findings are consistent with a pilomatricoma, a benign tumour of hair matrix origin. Pilomatricomas typically present as firm, subcutaneous nodules, often in the head and neck region. Cytology findings that include hair matrix-like cells and eosinophilic, anucleated cells (ghost cells) are characteristic of this tumour type.

The recommended approach is excisional biopsy, particularly through an upper blepharoplasty incision for lesions in the eyebrow area. This allows for both definitive diagnosis and complete removal while preserving local anatomy and achieving a favourable cosmetic outcome.

- **Core Biopsy** (Option B): Additional biopsy is unnecessary, as prior cytology has already suggested the diagnosis.
- **Incisional Biopsy** (Option C): While this could provide a partial tissue sample, it is inadequate for complete removal and definitive treatment.
- **Observation** (Option D): Observation is not ideal, as pilomatricomas tend to persist or enlarge.
- **Wide Local Excision with 5 mm Margins** (Option E): This is unnecessarily aggressive for a benign lesion without signs of malignancy. Such an approach would be destructive to the delicate anatomy of the eyebrow region, especially without a formal diagnosis or need for wide margins in benign lesions.

Q2. **Infantile haemangioma**

Answer: **D**. Surgical excision and laser therapy

Explanation: This patient's lesion is consistent with an infantile hemangioma (IH), a benign vascular tumour that typically appears within the first weeks of life, undergoes a phase of rapid growth (proliferation) for about nine months, and then gradually involutes, a process that is usually complete by 10–12 years of age. However, in some cases, IHs do not fully involute or respond to medical therapy.

Given that this hemangioma has not involuted spontaneously and has not responded to oral β-blocker therapy (atenolol), surgical excision combined with laser therapy is indicated. This approach is particularly appropriate due to the lesion's growth, proximity to the lower eyelid, and the potential for continued expansion, which could cause anatomical distortion or functional impairment if left untreated. Delaying treatment further may lead to more complex and destructive procedures in the future.

- **Intralesional Betamethasone (Option A)**: While corticosteroids were historically used, β-blockers have largely replaced them, and intralesional injections would be less effective given the lesion's size and location.
- **Observation (Option B)**: Observation is not suitable here, as the hemangioma has persisted beyond the typical involution age and is near the eye, posing a risk to function and anatomy.
- **Oral Propranolol (Option C)**: Although propranolol is effective for many hemangiomas, this lesion has already been unresponsive to a similar β-blocker (atenolol) and is unlikely to regress further.
- **Systemic Corticosteroids (Option E)**: Corticosteroids were previously used for IHs but are now generally reserved for cases unresponsive to β-blockers, and they carry significant side effects, especially in a paediatric population.

Q3. **Scar revision**

Answer: E. Z-plasty

Explanation: Z-plasty is a surgical technique that allows for scar revision by rearranging tissue to lengthen the scar and reduce tension, which can help improve contour and alignment, particularly in scars that cause contracture or distortion of natural anatomy, as in this case with the lip margin.

- **Chemical Peel (Option A)**: Primarily targets superficial discoloration or fine textural changes but will not correct the underlying contracture or margin distortion.
- **Dermabrasion (Option B)**: Can improve superficial texture but does not release scar contracture, which is necessary to restore normal lip contour.
- **Laser Therapy (Option C)**: Effective for colour and minor textural changes but does not alter the structural alignment or release contractures.
- **Skin Bleaching Agents (Option D)**: These may reduce pigmentation but will not affect the texture, contour, or structural distortion of the scar.

Q4. **Bilobed flap**

Answer: D. Bilobed flap

Explanation: For a full-thickness defect near the alar rim, a bilobed flap is an excellent choice. The bilobed flap allows for redistribution of nearby skin with similar characteristics, resulting in a more natural and aesthetically pleasing outcome. In this case, cartilage support is not necessary, so a composite graft is not required. Additionally, split-thickness or preauricular grafts are less suited for nasal reconstruction because of texture and thickness differences. Nasolabial flaps are typically reserved for larger defects.

Q5. **Management of lesions of the upper eyelid**

Answer: A. Direct closure of the defect

Explanation: For small upper eyelid defects that measure less than 25% of the horizontal dimension, direct closure is typically the best option, especially in elderly patients with some degree of lid laxity. In this case, the lid margin is preserved, and the tarsal plate is intact, making direct closure both feasible and appropriate. Larger defects greater than 25% may require lateral cantholysis with medial transposition, while defects approaching 60% often require a lid switch procedure. Extensive defects over 60% may call for a more complex reconstruction, such as a Cutler-Beard flap or Mustardé total lid flap. Local flaps like the nasolabial flap are less commonly used for small eyelid defects and are generally reserved for larger periorbital defects.

Q6. **Infectious causes of skin lesionst**

Answer: C. Sporothrix schenckii

Explanation: Sporothrix schenckii, a fungus associated with soil, plants, and decaying organic matter, causes sporotrichosis, commonly affecting gardeners (sometimes called rosepickers disease). The cutaneous form presents as a nodule that ulcerates, often with regional lymphadenopathy. Borrelia burgdorferi causes Lyme disease, characterised by erythema migrans rather than ulceration. Bacillus anthracis causes cutaneous anthrax, presenting with a black eschar and surrounding edema. Streptococcus pyogenes causes cellulitis or erysipelas, which typically lack ulceration. Rickettsia rickettsii, responsible for Rocky Mountain spotted fever, presents with a petechial or maculopapular rash, not ulceration.

Q7. **Infectious causes of skin lesions**

Answer: B. Poxvirus

Explanation: Molluscum contagiosum virus is a type of poxvirus. It typically presents as multiple small, umbilicated papules, commonly seen in children or immunosuppressed individuals. Human papillomavirus causes warts, which are verrucous and non-umbilicated. Herpes simplex virus and varicella-zoster virus cause vesicular lesions, not dome-shaped papules. Coxsackievirus causes hand-foot-and-mouth disease with vesicular lesions.

Q8. **Merkel cell carcinoma**

Answer: C. Merkel cell polyomavirus

Explanation: Merkel cell carcinoma is an aggressive neuroendocrine skin cancer strongly associated with Merkel cell polyomavirus. This virus integrates into the host genome, driving tumour progression. Epstein-Barr virus is linked to nasopharyngeal carcinoma and certain lymphomas. Human herpes virus 8 is associated with Kaposi sarcoma, which classically presents as flat, painless patches or nodules on the skin that are red, purple, bluish, brownish, or black.

Q9. **Merkel cell carcinoma**

Answer: B. Wide local excision with sentinel lymph node biopsy and adjuvant radiotherapy

Explanation: Merkel cell carcinoma is an aggressive neuroendocrine skin cancer with a high risk of metastasis and mortality. Management involves wide local excision with 1–2 cm margins, coupled with sentinel lymph node biopsy to evaluate regional spread. Adjuvant radiotherapy to the primary site and nodal basin reduces the risk of recurrence. Primary radiotherapy is reserved for patients who cannot undergo surgery. Chemotherapy is used for systemic disease, while immunotherapy with avelumab is specifically indicated for metastatic or inoperable cases.

Q10. **Margins for cutaneous SCC**

Answer: B. Surgical excision with a 6 mm margin

Explanation: High-risk cutaneous SCCs, such as those greater than 2 cm in size and located on the ear, require surgical excision with a margin of at least 6 mm for clear cancer clearance. NCCN Guidelines recommend excision with a 4 mm clinical margin for low-risk cSCC and wider (> 6 mm) clinical margin for high-risk cSCC tumours.

Q11. **Margins for cutaneous SCC**

Answer: C. Surgical excision with a 4 mm margin

Explanation: This lesion is considered a low-risk, well-defined cutaneous SCC. For low-risk tumours, surgical excision with a 4 mm margin provides a 95% clearance rate. High-risk features, such as large size (>2 cm), poor differentiation, or perineural invasion, are not present in this case. Therefore, surgical excision with a 4 mm margin is the treatment of choice.

Q12. **Gorlin-Goltz syndrome**

Answer: C. Nevoid basal cell carcinoma syndrome

Explanation: Gorlin-Goltz syndrome (also known as nevoid basal cell carcinoma syndrome) is an autosomal dominant condition characterised by multiple BCCs, palmar pitting, keratinising odontogenic cysts (often found in the jaw), and other features such as calcification of the falx cerebri, fused or bifid ribs, and cataracts. The presence of multiple BCCs, along with palmar pitting and a mandibular cyst, is highly suggestive of this syndrome.

Q13. **Mohs micrographic surgery**

Answer: D. Mohs micrographic surgery

Explanation: The British Association of Dermatologists (BAD) state for primary morphoeic BCC, a 3 mm margin gives a clearance rate of only 66%, while a 5 mm margin achieves 82%, and 13 mm is required to reach 95% clearance. Given the recurrent nature of this case, Mohs surgery is the most effective treatment. It ensures minimal tissue loss while achieving maximal clearance, which is particularly important in cosmetically and functionally sensitive regions.

Q14. **Initial management of suspected melanoma**

Answer: B. Excision with a 2 mm margin

Explanation: Lesions suspicious for melanoma should be excisionally biopsied with a 2 mm clinical margin and a cuff of underlying fat. This approach provides the diagnosis, determines the lesion's depth, and helps guide further management, such as wide local excision or staging procedures like sentinel lymph node biopsy. If excision cannot be performed without reconstruction, a full-thickness incisional or punch biopsy (2–4 mm) from the most elevated or dermoscopically abnormal area is acceptable to confirm the diagnosis. However, reconstruction should be avoided at this stage to prevent compromising future melanoma management. Observation is inappropriate for potentially malignant lesions, and a wider margin is only applied after the diagnosis and depth have been confirmed.

Q15. **Breslow thickness**

Answer: C. Wide local excision with a 2–3 cm margin

Explanation: According to the 2010 British Association of Dermatologists (BAD) guidelines, melanoma excision margins depend on Breslow thickness. For melanomas with a Breslow thickness of 1–2 mm, the recommended margin is 1–2 cm, which offers optimal oncologic control with excellent survival rates (95%–100% 5-year survival). For Breslow thicknesses of 2.1–4 mm, a margin of 2–3 cm is recommended. Observation or Mohs surgery is not suitable for invasive melanoma, and narrower margins would risk incomplete excision.

Q16. **Management of melanoma with nodal disease in the neck**

Answer: C. Therapeutic lymphadenectomy of the cervical lymph nodes

Explanation: Confirmed nodal metastasis requires therapeutic lymphadenectomy for complete removal of involved nodes and local control. Immunotherapy and radiotherapy may be considered in an adjuvant setting but do not replace lymphadenectomy for macroscopic nodal disease.

Q17. **Viral skin lesions**

Answer: A. Oral valacyclovir and urgent ophthalmology referral

Explanation: The clinical presentation suggests herpes zoster ophthalmicus with potential eye involvement. Immediate antiviral therapy combined with urgent ophthalmologic evaluation is critical to prevent vision loss.

Q18. **Keratoacanthoma**

Answer: D. Wide local excision with histopathology

Explanation: The clinical and histological description suggests keratoacanthoma. However, wide local excision is the most appropriate management to exclude malignancy and to avoid potential transformation into SCC. Cryotherapy and curettage are insufficient for ensuring histological assessment, and radiotherapy is not indicated for benign lesions.

Q19. **Actinic keratosis**

Answer: B. Topical 5-fluorouracil

Explanation: Actinic keratosis (AK) is a premalignant lesion caused by chronic sun exposure, with a risk of progression to SCC. It presents as a scaly, erythematous patch, often on sun-exposed areas like the scalp, face, and hands. First-line treatment includes topical 5-fluorouracil, which selectively targets dysplastic cells, leading to their destruction. Alternative treatments include imiquimod, cryotherapy, or photodynamic therapy, depending on lesion size and patient factors. Observation alone is not recommended due to the risk of malignant transformation. Mohs surgery or wide excision is typically reserved for confirmed SCC rather than premalignant lesions, and sentinel lymph node biopsy is unnecessary for AK.

Q20. **Management of cutaneous squamous cell carcinoma (SCC)**

Answer: C. Wide local excision with adjuvant radiotherapy

Explanation: Perineural invasion is a high-risk feature in squamous cell carcinoma that necessitates aggressive management. National guidelines recommend wide local excision with adjuvant radiotherapy for local control in cases with high-risk features.

Q21. **Anticoagulation and skin surgery**

Answer: D. Stop rivaroxiban 2 days before surgery and 24–48 hours postoperatively.

Explanation: Management of anticoagulation in patients on dabigatran undergoing significant surgery depends on the bleeding risk of the procedure and the patient's renal function. Dabigatran clearance is renal-dependent, and in patients with CrCl of 30–50 mL/min, the half-life of dabigatran is prolonged to approximately 13–14 hours. For significant surgical procedures, dabigatran should generally be stopped 48 hours before surgery and restarted 24 hours post operatively when renal function is not impaired. In this case, the patient has moderate renal impairment (CKD 3A), and many trusts would advocate stopping dabigatran earlier to reduce bleeding risk. Check your local guidelines for advice. Restarting anticoagulation should occur only after achieving adequate hemostasis to minimise the risk of postoperative bleeding. Idarucizumab, a reversal agent for dabigatran, is reserved for emergencies (e.g., life-threatening bleeding or urgent procedures) and is not typically used for elective surgeries.

Q22. **Negative-pressure wound therapy**

Answer: B. The optimal pressure for wound healing using NPWT is approximately 125 mmHg with an alternating pressure cycle of 5 minutes suction followed by 2 minutes off.

Explanation: The optimal pressure for vacuum-assisted closure (VAC) therapy is typically set at 125 mmHg with an alternating pressure cycle. This cycling mechanism promotes wound healing through mechanisms such as macro deformation, micro deformation (which aids in cellular proliferation and angiogenesis), and the removal of excess exudate, all contributing to improved tissue regeneration and wound healing. VAC therapy can be used on exposed bone or tendons as long as proper precautions are taken to avoid direct contact and damage to these structures. Contraindications for negative-pressure wound therapy include; non-enteric and unexplored fistulas, necrotic (dead) tissue or eschar that has not been debrided, wounds due to malignancy. Rarely, complications may occur which may require discontinuation of negative-pressure wound therapy. These may include: Pressure necrosis from the tubing, growth of granulation tissue into the foam dressing, contact dermatitis due to the adhesive, and fistula formation.

5 Trauma

QUESTIONS

Q1. A 32-year-old male is taken to the operating theatre as an emergency following major facial trauma. He has sustained a Markowitz III nasoethmoidal fracture, and injury to the nasolacrimal duct is suspected. During surgery, what is the most appropriate management of the suspected lacrimal system injury?
   A. Immediate dacryocystorhinostomy to bypass the damaged system
   B. Observation and reassessment in six weeks for persistent epiphora
   C. Placement of a Mini Monoka monocanalicular stent for a simple canalicular laceration
   D. Primary suturing of the canaliculus without stenting
   E. Enucleation to prevent further complications

Q2. A 10-year-old child presents with a unilateral mandibular condyle fracture with significant occlusal disruption, including an open bite. What is the most appropriate initial management?
   A. Analgesia and early mobilisation in all planes of mandibular movement
   B. Immediate surgical reduction and fixation
   C. Immobilisation for seven days with analgesia, followed by early mobilisation
   D. Immobilisation for two weeks with active mobilisation thereafter
   E. Immobilisation for six weeks

Q3. A patient underwent open reduction and internal fixation (ORIF) for right zygomaticomaxillary complex fractures requiring extensive access. They are now complaining that the right side of their face appears sagging compared to the left. Which of the following is not a useful technique to minimise the risk of soft tissue malposition?
   A. Suture closure of the periosteum over the inferior orbital rim
   B. Refixation of the periosteum over the anterior zygoma to the inferior orbital rim
   C. Placement of repositioning sutures from the periosteum on the anterior face of the zygoma to the temple area
   D. Avoiding closure of periosteal incisions to allow natural healing
   E. Repositioning of muscular attachments, such as the zygomaticus major and minor, onto the zygoma

Q4. A 30-year-old male presents to the emergency department after a high-speed motor vehicle collision. He is alert, cooperative, and has neck pain. Initial examination shows no neurological deficits, but he is unable to actively rotate his neck 45° in either direction due to pain. According to the NICE guidelines, what is the most appropriate next step in his management?

DOI: 10.1201/9781003609308-6

A. Discharge with neck injury advice and follow-up
B. Perform an MRI of the cervical spine within 48 hours
C. Apply a Philadelphia collar and observe for 24 hours
D. Perform a CT cervical spine scan within one hour
E. Immediate referral to spinal surgery

Q5. A 70-year-old man presents to the emergency department after falling down a flight of stairs, hitting his head. He briefly lost consciousness at the scene, and on examination, he has a Glasgow Coma Scale (GCS) score of 15, no focal neurological deficit, and no signs of skull fracture. He reports retrograde amnesia for 40 minutes before the fall. What is the most appropriate next step in management?
A. Discharge with head injury advice
B. Perform an MRI of the head within one hour
C. Perform a CT head scan within one hour
D. Perform a CT head scan within eight hours
E. Observe in the emergency department for 24 hours

Q6. You are in the emergency theatre performing primary stabilisation surgery for a 36-year-old male involved in a high-velocity road traffic collision. He has a Le Fort 3 fracture pattern with significant soft tissue injury in the left periorbital area. During irrigation of the periorbital wounds, you notice a peaked left pupil. Which of the following is not correct regarding the management of this patient?
A. Immediate referral to an ophthalmologist required.
B. A Fox shield should be applied over the eye postoperatively.
C. Anti-emetics should be administered to prevent vomiting.
D. Prophylactic antibiotics, including vancomycin and ceftazidime, required.
E. A Valsalva manoeuvre is required at the end of the procedure to ensure adequate haemostasis prior to closure.

Q7. A 40-year-old male presents with a Henderson Type 6 zygomatic fracture. Which of the following is the most appropriate incision to access and repair this fracture?
A. Coronal incision
B. Transconjunctival incision
C. Intraoral (Keen's) incision
D. Subciliary incision
E. Gillies temporal approach

Q8. A 28-year-old male presents to the emergency department with a penetrating neck injury after being assaulted with a knife. On examination, he has subcutaneous emphysema and difficulty swallowing. According to Monson's classification, the injury is located in Zone II of the neck. Which of the following is the most appropriate next step in management?
A. Apply local anaesthesia and observe for 24 hours
B. Immediate explorative surgery
C. Remove any impaled object in the field to prevent further damage

D. Perform a CT angiogram before deciding on surgery
E. Discharge the patient with wound care instructions if the platysma is intact

Q9. A 35-year-old male presents to the emergency department 48 hours after a motor vehicle accident with facial trauma. He has ptosis, ophthalmoplegia, proptosis, and a fixed dilated pupil in the left eye. Examination reveals loss of the corneal reflex and decreased lacrimal secretion on the same side. CT imaging shows bony fragments near the superior orbital fissure. Which of the following is the most appropriate next step in management?
A. Canthotomy and cantholysis then repeat imaging in 48 hours
B. Observation and repeat imaging in 48 hours
C. Urgent surgical decompression in theatre
D. Arrange MRI of the brain to rule out intracranial pathology
E. Initiate high-dose steroids to reduce inflammation

Q10. A 40-year-old woman presents to the clinic with complaints of a sunken appearance on the left side of her forehead following a craniotomy performed six months ago. She reports feeling self-conscious due to the asymmetry and requests a solution for the indentation. Which of the following is the most appropriate management option?
A. Observation and reassurance that the hollowing will resolve spontaneously
B. Injection of botulinum toxin into the temporalis muscle
C. Surgical fat grafting to the affected area
D. Physical therapy and massage of the temporal region
E. High-dose corticosteroid injections to reduce hollowing

Q11. A 28-year-old male presents with jaw pain and difficulty chewing after being struck on the side of his face during a fight. Examination reveals lateral crossbite and tenderness over the coronoid process. Imaging confirms a linear fracture of the left coronoid process with mild displacement. The patient reports severe pain with mandibular movement. What is the most appropriate management?
A. Immediate intraoral open reduction and fixation
B. Removal of the fractured coronoid segment
C. Intermaxillary fixation in occlusion for three to four weeks
D. Conservative treatment with analgesia and mandibular exercises
E. Observation only without further intervention

Q12. A 30-year-old male with a mandibular condyle fracture is discussed at the trauma multi-disciplinary team (MDT) meeting and agreed for open reduction and internal fixation (ORIF). Which of the following is a relative indication for ORIF of the condyle?
A. Lateral extracapsular displacement of the condyle
B. Condylar displacement into the middle cranial fossa
C. Fragment angulation exceeding 10°
D. Inability to achieve adequate occlusion using closed reduction techniques
E. Invasion by a foreign body into the condylar region

Q13. A 65-year-old female with long-standing rheumatoid arthritis presents for emergency surgery. She has a fixed flexion deformity of the neck, and during induction of anaesthesia, the anaesthetist is unable to intubate or ventilate the patient. Oxygen saturation is rapidly falling. What is the most appropriate next step in airway management?

A. Perform a needle cricothyroidotomy
B. Attempt blind nasal intubation
C. Perform a surgical cricothyroidotomy
D. Reattempt intubation with a smaller endotracheal tube
E. Perform a tracheostomy in the operating room

Q14. A 6-year-old child presents after blunt neck trauma with obvious signs of laryngotracheal disruption, including subcutaneous emphysema and respiratory distress. Oxygen saturation is 88% and attempts to secure an airway via endotracheal intubation have failed. What is the most appropriate next step in airway management?

A. Perform needle cricothyroidotomy
B. Attempt bag-mask ventilation with positive pressure
C. Perform surgical tracheostomy under local anaesthesia
D. Reattempt intubation with a smaller endotracheal tube
E. Use a supraglottic airway device

Q15. A 4-year-old child is brought to the emergency department following a generalised tonic-clonic seizure. The child is unresponsive, with gurgling noises heard on respiration and oxygen saturation of 88%. What is the most appropriate immediate step in airway management?

A. Insert a nasopharyngeal airway and provide supplemental oxygen
B. Perform endotracheal intubation under sedation
C. Suction the airway and utilise a jaw thrust
D. Perform a surgical cricothyroidotomy
E. Use a bag-mask device to ventilate with positive pressure

Q16. A 28-year-old professional martial arts fighter presents with a saddle nose deformity following repeated trauma and ongoing episodes of epistaxis. Examination reveals nasal dorsum collapse, septal perforation, and widened nasal base. What is the most appropriate surgical management?

A. Closed reduction with septoplasty
B. Open reduction with dorsal graft reconstruction using autologous cartilage
C. Dorsal graft reconstruction with titanium mesh
D. Rhinoplasty with alloplastic implant augmentation
E. Endoscopic cauterisation of nasal vessels

Q17. A 45-year-old male presents with a supraorbital rim fracture following a road traffic accident. He has diplopia on upward gaze and a restricted upward gaze. CT imaging confirms impingement of the superior rectus muscle by bone fragments. What is the most appropriate surgical management?

A. Observation and regular follow-up
B. Open reduction and internal fixation via upper eyelid incision
C. Transcranial decompression of the orbital roof
D. Endoscopic removal of bone fragments with orbital roof repair
E. Open reduction and internal fixation with titanium plating via coronal incision

Q18. A 10-year-old child presents 24 hours after sustaining a nasal fracture from a fall. The fracture is minimally displaced with no nasal obstruction or septal hematoma. What is the most appropriate management?
  A. Immediate closed reduction under local anaesthesia
  B. Closed reduction under general anaesthesia within seven days
  C. Observation with nasal splint application
  D. Open reduction with internal fixation
  E. Referral to ENT for endoscopic nasal surgery

Q19. A 35-year-old male presents following a high-energy trauma to the glabella region. He has an open wound with flattening of the nasal bridge and telecanthus. CT confirms displaced nasoethmoidal fractures with significantly comminution of the left medial orbital wall. What is the most appropriate surgical management?
  A. Closed reduction with nasal splint
  B. Open reduction with internal fixation
  C. Open reduction with internal fixation plus canthopexy wire
  D. Initial wound washout and soft tissue repair with delayed open reduction internal fixation
  E. Initial wound washout and rhinoplasty with cartilage grafting

Q20. A 93-year-old presents with a large orbital floor fracture causing enophthalmos but no functional vision impairment. The patient has significant comorbidities including severe dementia requiring full time care and hoist for transfer. What is the most appropriate management?
  A. Orbital floor repair with stock titanium mesh
  B. Observation and reassurance
  C. Orbital decompression to prevent further complications
  D. Endoscopic repair of orbital floor
  E. Orbital floor repair with patient specific implant

Q21. A 33-year-old woman is reviewed in the clinic three months after emergency surgery for a road traffic collision involving penetrating trauma to the left side of the neck, pan-facial fractures, and injury to the left parotid duct. On examination, she has ptosis on the left, and her left pupil constricts in response to light but dilates very slowly after the light is removed. Which of the following is correct?
  A. Symptoms are due to compression of the oculomotor nerve (CN III)
  B. The patient likely has an injury to the left cavernous sinus
  C. Her presentation is due to a carotid artery dissection
  D. This condition will resolve spontaneously within a few weeks
  E. Her symptoms are explained by facial nerve injury which was missed when repairing the parotid duct.

Q22. A 27-year-old male presents after a stab wound to the cheek in the region of the midpupillary line. On examination, there is slight asymmetry and weakness on smiling.
Which of the following muscles is most likely injured?

A. Risorius
B. Zygomaticus major
C. Orbicularis oris
D. Levator labii superioris
E. Buccinator

Q23. A 35-year-old male with a large frontal skull defect following trauma is scheduled for cranioplasty using a custom alloplastic implant. Which of the following advantages best supports the use of alloplastic materials over autologous grafts in this scenario?
A. Reduced risk of infection compared to autologous materials
B. Ability to provide precise contouring and aesthetic reconstruction
C. Superior integration with native bone and surrounding tissue
D. Lower risk of long-term material resorption or failure
E. Minimised operative time due to pre-surgical graft preparation

Q24. A 42-year-old woman undergoes tissue expansion for scalp reconstruction following a burn injury. During the expansion process, the patient develops localised erythema and discomfort at the expansion site. Which of the following best explains the primary physiological adaptations occurring during successful tissue expansion?
A. Fibroblast-mediated deposition of mature collagen bundles with reduced vascularity
B. Recruitment of stem cells and inflammatory cytokines from the periphery of the expander
C. Mechanical stretch stimulating neovascularisation and extracellular matrix remodelling
D. Compensatory dermal hypertrophy with elastin fibre fragmentation
E. Epidermal thinning and dermal ischaemia at the leading edge of the expander

Q25. A 32-year-old male undergoes open reduction and internal fixation of a mandibular fracture. Which process is primarily responsible for healing under rigid fixation?
A. Endochondral ossification
B. Intramembranous ossification
C. Woven bone formation
D. Fibrocartilaginous callus formation
E. Bone remodelling

Q26. A 40-year-old male presents with a depressed frontal sinus fracture. CT imaging shows comminution and involvement of the 30% of the posterior table but no CSF leak. The patient's medical history includes Addison's disease and Type 2 diabetes. What is the most appropriate initial management?
A. Observation and serial imaging
B. Immediate sinus obliteration with fat graft
C. Open reduction and internal fixation with cranialisation of the sinus
D. Craniotomy and dural repair
E. Endoscopic repair of the sinus fracture

Q27. A 38-year-old male with suspected pan-facial fractures develops severe haemorrhage from the oral cavity. The ED team have been unable to control the bleeding. What is the most appropriate next step in management?

A. Perform immediate maxillomandibular fixation
B. Pack the oral cavity and perform endotracheal intubation
C. Immediate embolisation of the maxillary artery
D. Administer intravenous tranexamic acid
E. Perform nasal intubation and perform external carotid artery ligation

Q28. A 25-year-old male with multiple injuries from a road traffic accident is diagnosed with a significant haemorrhage from a left body of mandibular fracture and Le Fort II fractures. Primary survey also reveals suspected pelvic fracture, possible bladder rupture, left pneumothorax and left upper limb lacerations. What is the most important next step in this patient's management?

A. Reduction of mandibular fracture
B. Temporary stabilisation of Le Fort fracture
C. Needle thoracostomy
D. Urethral catheter
E. Placement of pelvic binder

Q29. A 40-year-old male presents 24 hours after being struck in the face by a metal bar. He has periorbital bruising, infraorbital numbness, and limited upward gaze. A CT scan reveals a comminuted orbital floor fracture with herniation of orbital contents into the maxillary sinus. Four days later, he returns with worsening diplopia, periorbital swelling, and a fever of 38.2°C. What is the most appropriate management option?

A. Immediate surgical decompression of the orbit
B. Broad-spectrum intravenous antibiotics and hospitalisation
C. High-dose intravenous corticosteroids
D. Delayed orbital floor repair after resolution of infection
E. Nasal decongestants with outpatient follow-up

Q30. A 10-year-old boy presents to the emergency department after being struck in the face by a baseball. He complains of pain around his eye and has nausea, vomiting, and bradycardia. On examination, he has limited upward gaze and periorbital swelling, but no obvious external trauma. What is the next step in managing this patient?

A. Observation with follow-up in one week
B. Administration of intravenous corticosteroids
C. CT scan of the orbit followed by conservative management
D. CT scan of the orbit and urgent surgical intervention
E. CT scan of the orbit with delayed surgical intervention if symptoms persist

Q31. A 22-year-old male presents to the A&E with facial burns following a kitchen accident where hot oil splashed onto his face. On examination, the patient exhibits the following:

- Red, swollen skin with blistering over the cheek and forehead.
- The burn is painful but there is no loss of sensation.
- The skin blanches on pressure but takes longer to return to its normal colour.

Which of the following statements is true?

A. Immediate surgical excision of the burned tissue is recommended to reduce the risk of scarring and promote faster healing.
B. The patient should be started on intralesional corticosteroids as part of the initial treatment to minimise the risk of hypertrophic scarring.
C. Topical antibiotic ointments should be applied to prevent infection.
D. These burns usually heal within two to three weeks with minimal risk of significant scarring.
E. Early full thickness skin grafting is often required to minimise long-term sequelae.

Q32. A 35-year-old male presents to the emergency department three weeks after sustaining severe cranio-orbital trauma in a road traffic accident. He reports progressive worsening of eye symptoms, including bulging of his left eye, redness, and visual disturbance. On examination, you note:

- Pulsatile exophthalmos of the left eye.
- Marked chemosis and proptosis.
- A dilated, non-reactive pupil on the affected side.
- Ophthalmoplegia with restricted extraocular movements.
- An audible bruit heard over the left orbit.

Contrast-enhanced CT reveals arterialisation of the superior ophthalmic vein.
Which of the following is the most appropriate treatment for this condition?

A. High-dose corticosteroids to reduce inflammation and prevent optic nerve compression.
B. Surgical decompression of the superior orbital fissure to relieve pressure.
C. Endovascular embolisation to restore normal vascular anatomy and flow.
D. Observation and follow-up as the condition typically resolves spontaneously.
E. External beam radiotherapy to reduce vascular engorgement and improve symptoms.

Q33. A 45-year-old male presents with traumatic facial injuries following a road traffic accident. Imaging reveals multiple fractures of the lateral orbital wall and floor, with herniation of orbital fat into adjacent fossae. During surgical exploration, the surgeon relies on deep orbital landmarks for safe dissection and reconstruction.
Which of the following statements is true?

A. The infraorbital nerve lies superficial to the floor of the orbit throughout its entire course.
B. The trigone of the greater wing of the sphenoid is uniformly thick and rarely fractured.
C. The orbital plate of the palatine bone is a weak structure prone to disruption in blunt trauma.
D. Division of the contents of the inferior orbital fissure is safe, as no critical neurovascular structures pass through it.
E. The deep orbit commences at the 1.5 cm deep to the infraorbital rim.

ANSWERS AND EXPLANATIONS

Q1. **Nasolacrimal duct injury**

Answer: C. Placement of a Mini Monoka monocanalicular stent for a simple canalicular laceration

Explanation: In cases of nasolacrimal duct injury associated with facial trauma, prompt exploration and repair are crucial to preserving tear drainage and preventing chronic epiphora. A Mini Monoka monocanalicular stent is an effective option for simple monocanalicular injuries (8), while more complex bicanalicular lacerations may require bicanalicular stents such as Crawford or Ritleng tubes. These stents typically remain in place for 8–12 weeks to maintain duct patency. Delayed intervention or observation risks canalicular obstruction and persistent tearing, and primary suturing alone is inadequate due to the delicate structure of the lacrimal drainage system. Dacryocystorhinostomy is only indicated for chronic obstruction, and enucleation is not a relevant management strategy in this scenario.

Q2. **Paediatric mandibular condyle fractures**

Answer: D. Immobilisation for two weeks followed by early mobilisation

Explanation: In paediatric patients under 12 years old, most mandibular condyle fractures can heal with minimal intervention due to the high remodelling potential. Much disagreement exists in the literature for optimal management of paediatric condyle fractures. Primarily, this is due to risks associated with both IMF and ORIF including iatrogenic injury to teeth and nerves, as well as ankylosis. However, in cases of significant occlusal disruption, such as with an open bite following a unilateral condyle fracture, closed reduction and a period of immobilisation for two weeks is often recommended to allow for proper healing and occlusal alignment. After this period, early mobilisation is important to minimise ankylosis risk and maintain mandibular function (9). Surgery is typically reserved for severe cases or failures of conservative treatment. Longer periods of immobilisation are generally indicated for bilateral fractures or older adolescents.

Q3. **Soft tissue resuspension in midface trauma**

Answer: D. Avoiding closure of periosteal incisions to allow natural healing

Explanation: Avoiding closure of periosteal incisions is **not** a useful technique and may increase the risk of soft tissue malposition. Proper closure and refixation of the periosteum, particularly over the inferior orbital rim and the anterior zygoma, are essential steps to ensure soft tissue is correctly aligned over the bony structures following surgery. Techniques such as repositioning sutures to the temple area and reattaching muscular attachments (e.g., zygomaticus major and minor) onto the zygoma help to support and stabilise the soft tissue, preventing sagging or diastasis.

Q4. **Management of C-spine injuries**

Answer: D. Perform a CT cervical spine scan within one hour

Explanation: According to NICE guidelines, a CT cervical spine scan should be performed within 1 hour for patients aged 16 and over with a head or neck injury and specific risk factors. In this case, the patient has experienced a dangerous mechanism of injury (high-speed motor vehicle collision) and is unable to actively rotate his neck 45° in both directions due to pain. These factors warrant a prompt CT cervical spine scan to assess for potential cervical spine injury. Discharging the patient, observing without imaging, or opting for MRI rather than CT does not align with the guidelines for managing potential cervical spine injuries in this context.

Q5. **Management of C-spine injuries**

Answer: D. Perform a CT head scan within eight hours

Explanation: According to NICE guidelines, a CT head scan should be performed within 8 hours for patients aged 16 and over with a head injury who have experienced some loss of consciousness or amnesia, if they also meet any additional risk factors. This patient is over 65 years old and has more than 30 minutes of retrograde amnesia, both of which meet the criteria for a CT head scan within 8 hours. MRI is not recommended as the primary imaging modality for detecting acute traumatic brain injury, and immediate CT within 1 hour is reserved for patients with more urgent risk factors (e.g., GCS <15 at 2 hours post-injury, suspected skull fracture, post-traumatic seizure). Discharge or observation alone would not be appropriate given the risk factors present.

Q6. **Globe rupture**

Answer: E. A Valsalva manoeuvre is required at the end of the procedure to ensure adequate haemostasis prior to closure.

Explanation: Performing a Valsalva manoeuvre in this context is **incorrect** as it would increase intraocular pressure, which could worsen the injury and potentially lead to herniation of ocular contents. A peaked pupil in this setting raises concern for a possible globe rupture, requiring immediate referral to an ophthalmologist for urgent intervention. Correct management includes protecting the eye with a Fox shield to prevent external pressure, administering anti-emetics to reduce intraocular pressure from vomiting, and providing prophylactic antibiotics (such as vancomycin and ceftazidime) to prevent post-traumatic endophthalmitis. Assessing and updating tetanus status is also recommended in cases of traumatic injury.

Q7. **Henderson classification**

Answer: B. Transconjunctival incision

Explanation: A Henderson Type 6 fracture involves only the orbital rim, and the transconjunctival incision is commonly used to access the orbital rim and floor with minimal visible scarring. This approach provides good exposure to the orbital rim while avoiding a visible scar on the lower eyelid. A subciliary incision could also provide access to the orbital rim but may carry a higher risk of visible scarring or lower eyelid malposition. A bicoronal incision is more invasive and typically reserved for more complex fractures or those involving the zygomatic arch and frontal region. The intraoral (Keen's) incision is used for fractures of the zygomatic arch or body but does not provide adequate access to the orbital rim. The Gillies temporal approach is used primarily for zygomatic arch fractures.

Q8. **Penetrating neck injury**

Answer: B. Immediate explorative surgery

Explanation: This patient presents with "hard signs" of penetrating neck injury, including subcutaneous emphysema and difficulty swallowing, which indicate a potential airway or vascular injury. In the presence of hard signs (such as shock, pulsatile bleeding, expanding hematoma, airway compromise, and subcutaneous emphysema), immediate explorative surgery is recommended to address potentially life-threatening injuries. Observing the patient or performing imaging (e.g., CT angiogram) may delay critical intervention. Impaled objects should not be removed in the field, as this can exacerbate bleeding or other injuries. If the platysma is intact, the wound is considered superficial, but in this case, the the presence of subcutaneous emphysema mandates urgent surgical intervention.

Q9. **Superior orbital fissure syndrome**

Answer: C. Urgent surgical decompression

Explanation: This patient presents with classic features of superior orbital fissure syndrome following trauma, including ptosis, ophthalmoplegia, proptosis, a fixed dilated pupil, and sensory deficits in the distribution of the ophthalmic division of the trigeminal nerve (e.g., loss of corneal reflex and lacrimal hyposecretion). Superior orbital fissure syndrome is a medical emergency, and if orbitocranial trauma is the cause, urgent surgical decompression is necessary to relieve pressure on the neurovascular structures and improve prognosis. Observation or delayed imaging would not be appropriate given the risk of permanent neurological damage. MRI is useful in non-traumatic cases but less valuable here, as CT has already identified bony fragments. Lubricating eye drops alone are insufficient, as they do not address the underlying cause. High-dose steroids may reduce inflammation but are not a substitute for decompression in trauma-induced superior orbital fissure syndrome.

Q10. **Temporal hollowing**

Answer: C. Surgical fat grafting to the affected area

Explanation: Temporal hollowing is a common cosmetic and functional concern following craniotomy or trauma due to atrophy or detachment of the temporalis muscle and loss of soft tissue volume. The most effective treatment is often surgical fat grafting, which can restore volume and improve symmetry by filling the hollowed area. Other options include implant placement or repositioning of temporalis muscle. High-dose corticosteroid injections are not indicated, as they could exacerbate atrophy and worsen the appearance.

Q11. **Coronoid fractures**

Answer: C. Intermaxillary fixation in occlusion for three to four weeks

Explanation: In cases of coronoid fractures with severe pain or significant malocclusion, intermaxillary fixation (IMF) for three to four weeks is the most appropriate treatment. IMF helps to stabilise the fracture, reduce pain, and allow for proper healing by splinting the fractured segment. Conservative treatment with analgesia and exercises is adequate for minimally symptomatic or non-displaced fractures, but in this case, the patient's symptoms and malocclusion warrant more active management. Surgical interventions, such as open reduction or coronoid segment removal, are reserved for cases with impaired mandibular function due to large fractures or fibrosis of the temporalis muscle. Observation alone is not sufficient for this presentation, as the malocclusion and severe pain need to be addressed.

Q12. **Condyle fractures**

Answer: C. Fragment angulation exceeding 10°

Explanation: Absolute indications for open reduction and internal fixation (ORIF) of mandibular condyle fractures were first proposed by Zide and Kent in

1983. These include displacement of the condyle into the middle cranial fossa, condylar fractures with foreign body invasion, and inability to achieve proper occlusion using closed reduction techniques. Relative indications, such as fragment angulation exceeding 10°, may impair mandibular function and warrant surgical intervention to restore anatomy. The decision for ORIF considers fracture severity, functional demands, and the need to minimise long-term complications like ankylosis or malocclusion balanced against the risks which the patient must be fully informed of.

Q13. **Surgical airway**

Answer: C. Perform a surgical cricothyroidotomy

Explanation: In a "cannot intubate, cannot ventilate" (CICV) scenario, a surgical cricothyroidotomy is the most appropriate immediate intervention to establish a secure airway and restore oxygenation. Difficult Airway Society (DAS) 2015 guidelines (https://das.uk.com/guidelines/das_intubation_guidelines/) recommend cricothyroidotomy first and then progressing to tracheostomy once the airway is secured. Needle cricothyroidotomy is also a suitable option, but access will need conversion to a larger diameter inlet/outlet rapidly or else ventilation becomes ineffective, and jet ventilators are not always available.

Q14. **Surgical airway**

Answer: C. Perform surgical tracheostomy under local anaesthesia

Explanation: In cases of suspected laryngotracheal disruption, surgical tracheostomy is the preferred approach to bypass the disrupted airway and secure ventilation. All other options are unlikely to be successful due to the level of disruption. For a CICV scenario for a paediatric patient with normal airway anatomy, it is worth noting two conflicting guidelines given the rarity of the scenario. DAS guidelines 2015 advocate for needle cricothyroidotomy first line if <8 years of age with scalpel techniques second line if needle techniques fail. If the patient is >8 years of age, a scalpel technique is advocated for all front of neck access. In contrast, Advanced Paediatric Life Support (APLS) suggests that needle techniques should only be attempted in children over the age of 5 years with scalpel techniques preferred in those <5 years (via tracheostomy in <1 year and cricothyroidotomy or tracheostomy in 1- to 5-year-olds).

Q15. **Airway manoeuvres**

Answer: C. Suction the airway and utilise a jaw thrust

Explanation: In post-seizure patients, airway compromise is often caused by secretions or tongue obstruction. Clearance/suctioning removes secretions, and a jaw thrust can help to reposition the tongue for better ventilation whilst keeping c-spine neutral. Intubation is not immediately indicated unless there is continued airway compromise or recurrent seizures. Airway adjuncts such as a nasopharyngeal airway may be appropriate as a next step. Surgical interventions and bag-mask ventilation are unnecessary unless ventilation is inadequate after simpler measures.

Q16. **Traumatic saddle nose deformity**

Answer: B. Open reduction with dorsal graft reconstruction using autologous cartilage

Explanation: A saddle nose deformity caused by repetitive trauma requires open reduction and reconstruction with dorsal grafts, often using autologous cartilage (e.g., from the rib or ear) to restore the nasal dorsum and septum while preventing long-term complications.

Q17. **Orbital fractures**

Answer: E. Open reduction and internal fixation with titanium plating via coronal incision

Explanation: A supraorbital rim fracture with eye signs such as diplopia and muscle impingement requires open reduction and internal fixation to relieve impingement and restore orbital anatomy. This may be possible with a patient specific implant. In order to obtain adequate access to the roof of the orbit, a coronal incision is likely required. Observation is inappropriate due to functional impairment. Transcranial decompression is not required unless there is significant intracranial involvement. Endoscopic approaches are not feasible for this fracture location.

Q18. **Nasal bone fracture management**

Answer: C. Observation with nasal splint application

Explanation: Minimally displaced nasal fractures in children are typically managed conservatively with observation and splinting, as significant remodelling often occurs naturally. Closed reduction would be of benefit for displaced fractures. Open reduction is unnecessary in this context. Endoscopic surgery is not indicated without functional impairment or obstruction.

Q19. **Naso-orbitoethmoid (NOE) fractures**

Answer: C. Open reduction with internal fixation plus canthopexy wire

Explanation: NOE fractures often occur as part of a broader pan-facial injury, and proper reduction of each element is crucial for overall restoration. The frontal nasal angle should be corrected by reducing the fracture and stabilising it with low-profile plates. In cases of severe comminution, primary bone grafting with split calvarium may be necessary. Accurate reduction of the central fragment, which is frequently impacted, is essential. Medial orbital wall defects can be repaired using adaptive titanium plates placed from the orbital side. Treatment varies based on Markowitz classification, with type 1 injuries requiring no additional stabilisation of the medial canthal ligament, while types 2 and 3 necessitate identification of the ligament using specialised canthopexy wires.

Q20. **Orbital floor fracture management**

Answer: B. Observation and reassurance

Explanation: In an elderly, immobile patient with severe dementia and no functional vision impairment, observation and reassurance are the most appropriate management. Surgery will be of limited benefit to quality of life and has significant risks.

Q21. **Horner's syndrome**

Answer: C. These findings are consistent with Horner's syndrome caused by a carotid artery dissection

Explanation: Horner's syndrome is caused by disruption of the sympathetic nervous system pathway, resulting in ptosis, miosis (pupillary constriction), and anhidrosis. In this patient, the slow dilation of the left pupil after light is removed suggests sympathetic dysfunction.

In cases of neck trauma, carotid artery dissection is a common cause of Horner's syndrome, as the sympathetic fibres run along the wall of the internal carotid artery. This condition does not involve the oculomotor nerve (CN III), which controls extra-ocular movements and is associated with complete pupillary dilation in its dysfunction.

Q22. **Mimetic musculature**

Answer: D. Levator labii superioris

Explanation: Several mimetic muscles are important for co-ordinated movements to produce a variety of smile types. The levator labii superioris muscle is involved in elevating the upper lip. A stab wound in the midpupillary line would likely affect this muscle, resulting in slight asymmetry and weakness on smiling. Zygomaticus major is also involved in elevation of the upper lip and lateral movement, which is important in smiling. The risorius controls facial expressions of lateral movement (smiling and laughing), but it would not primarily cause weakness in upper lip elevation. The orbicularis oris and buccinator muscles play roles in lip closure and cheek compression.

Q23. **Alloplastic implants**

Answer: B. Ability to provide precise contouring and aesthetic reconstruction

Explanation: Alloplastic materials, particularly custom-designed implants, allow for precise contouring to restore cranial aesthetics and symmetry. While they have certain disadvantages, such as a higher infection risk compared to autologous grafts, their ability to achieve superior aesthetic outcomes in cases of large or complex defects makes them ideal for cranioplasty in this scenario.

Q24. **Tissue expansion**

Answer: C. Mechanical stretch stimulating neovascularisation and extracellular matrix remodelling

Explanation: Tissue expansion relies on mechanical stretch, which triggers cellular proliferation, angiogenesis, and remodelling of the extracellular matrix to generate additional skin. While fibroblast activity, cytokine recruitment, and localised hypertrophic responses may contribute, they are not the primary mechanism. Thinning and ischaemia represent complications rather than physiological adaptations.

Q25. **Mandibular fracture healing**

Answer: B. Intramembranous ossification

Explanation: The mandible forms via intramembranous ossification. However, current research shows, similar to long bones, it heals with a combination of intramembranous and endochondral ossification. Cartilage formation and endochondral repair is favoured if there is a high amount of mechanical motion between the fracture ends. Rigid fixation allows direct bone healing via intramembranous ossification without the formation of a cartilaginous callus.

Q26. **Management of frontal sinus fractures**

Answer: C. Open reduction and internal fixation with cranialisation of the sinus

Explanation: Severe fractures which result in disruption of greater than 25% of the posterior table should be considered for cranialisation. This is to prevent complications like meningitis or brain abscess, particularly in immunocompromised patients such as this. If fit and well, a small undisplaced fracture of the posterior table may be suitable for observation and appropriate antimicrobial cover alone pending discussion with neurosurgery.

Q27. **Control of haemorrhage**

Answer: B. Pack the oral cavity and perform endotracheal intubation

Explanation: Life-threatening oral cavity haemorrhage requires several early critical steps and should be managed in an appropriate setting. Using an A–E approach, secure a definitive airway early and control haemorrhage. Bite-blocks should be available in Resus in the emergency department. If endotracheal intubation is not possible then follow the difficult airway guidelines and consider cricothyroidotomy. Local major haemorrhage protocols should be followed for resuscitation with appropriate fluids early on.

Q28. **Management of pneumothorax**

Answer: C. Needle thoracostomy

Explanation: In a multiply-injured patient, management follows ATLS principles. Airway, breathing, and circulation take precedence, making treatment of pneumothorax the immediate priority over the other injuries. Haemorrhage from bony injuries can be controlled with stabilisation prior to definitive management.

Q29. **Orbital cellulitis**

Answer: A. Immediate surgical decompression of the orbit

Explanation: The patient is showing signs of orbital cellulitis, which requires urgent treatment with broad-spectrum intravenous antibiotics and surgical drainage to prevent vision loss. Surgical decompression is necessary given the worsening diplopia. Corticosteroids are not recommended during active infection, and nasal decongestants alone are insufficient to manage orbital cellulitis.

Q30. **White eye blow-out fracture**

Answer: D. CT scan of the orbit and urgent surgical intervention

Explanation: This child likely has a trapdoor fracture, which is common in paediatric patients and can lead to muscle entrapment, resulting in the oculocardiac reflex (nausea, vomiting, bradycardia). Urgent surgical intervention is required to release the entrapped muscle and prevent further systemic complications while restoring normal ocular movement. Delaying surgery could lead to long-term ocular dysfunction, including persistent diplopia or loss of binocular vision.

Q31. **Burns**

Answer: D. These burns usually heal within 2–3 weeks with minimal risk of significant scarring.

Explanation: The patient's presentation is consistent with a superficial dermal (partial thickness) burn, which affects the epidermis and the upper layers of the dermis. These burns typically present as red, swollen skin with blistering, and are painful but without loss of sensation. Capillary refill blanches but takes longer to return to normal, reflecting damage to the dermal capillaries. Superficial dermal burns generally heal within two to three weeks with appropriate wound care. Management techniques include maintaining a moist environment, preventing infection, and avoiding excessive tension on the skin. Immediate surgical excision, intralesional corticosteroids, or early skin grafting are not indicated for these burns, as they usually heal on their own with conservative treatment. Topical antibiotics may be advocated by some, but they are not currently supported by NICE for first line management.

Q32. **Caroticocavernous fistula (CCF)**

Answer: C. Endovascular embolisation to restore normal vascular anatomy and flow.

Explanation: The patient presents with clinical features consistent with a CCF, including pulsatile exophthalmos, chemosis, proptosis, cranial nerve disruption (ophthalmoplegia and a dilated pupil), and an audible bruit, with diagnosis confirmed by arterialisation of the superior ophthalmic vein on contrast CT. The most appropriate treatment is endovascular embolisation, which restores normal vascular flow and prevents complications such as vision loss or further cranial nerve dysfunction. Other options are incorrect: high-dose corticosteroids may be used as an adjunct in orbital compartment syndrome but not for vascular anomalies, like CCF. Surgical intervention may be required but decompression alone will not treat the cause. Observation is inappropriate given the level of symptoms but may be suitable for very small CCF. External beam radiotherapy is more appropriate for conditions like orbital tumours (10).

Q33. **Anatomy of the deep orbit**

Answer: D. Division of the contents of the inferior orbital fissure is safe, as no critical neurovascular structures pass through it.

Explanation: The deep orbit commences at the anterior edge of the inferior orbital fissure. The trigone of the greater wing of the sphenoid is a robust part of the lateral orbital wall that separates the orbit from the middle cranial fossa. While most fractures of the greater wing involve the thinner anterolateral portion, displaced fractures of the trigone are rare but can compress the optic nerve, potentially causing sudden and irreversible vision loss. The infraorbital nerve runs beneath the orbital floor and becomes superficial posteriorly, serving as an important surgical landmark but making the statement about it being entirely superficial incorrect. The orbital plate of the palatine bone is a strong and reliable structure in the deep orbit that resists blunt trauma; as such, it is a useful landmark for positioning implants to reconstruct the orbital floor. Although the inferior orbital fissure does not transmit critical neurovascular structures, surgical dissection still requires care to preserve adjacent important structures like the infraorbital nerve and ophthalmic vein (11).

6 Salivary Gland

QUESTIONS

Q1. A 46-year-old woman with systemic lupus erythematosus presents with persistent dry mouth and dry eyes. She has had these symptoms for over six months, and recent examination reveals bilateral lacrimal gland swelling. Lab results show positive anti-Ro/SS-A and anti-La/SS-B antibodies, along with reduced unstimulated salivary flow rate. Which of the following should be done next to confirm the diagnosis?

A. Salivary scintigraphy
B. Schirmer test
C. Rose Bengal Score for corneal ulceration
D. Lower labial gland biopsy
E. Serum antinuclear antibody test

Q2. A 60-year-old man with primary Sjögren's syndrome presents with new unilateral parotid gland enlargement and associated fatigue, low-grade fever, and weight loss over the past month. Imaging of the parotid gland reveals a single hypoechoic lesion in the parotid tail with irregular borders. Two prior ultrasound guided fine-needle aspirations have been attempted and were inconclusive. What is the most appropriate next step in management?

A. Serial ultrasound imaging
B. Initiate high-dose corticosteroids
C. Sialography for further structural assessment
D. Open parotid biopsy of the lesion
E. Start symptomatic treatment with pilocarpine

Q3. A 45-year-old man presents with a painless, ballotable swelling over his right parotid region ten days after undergoing a parotidectomy. Examination reveals clear fluid draining through a small skin defect. Fluid analysis shows elevated amylase levels. Aspiration was performed twice, but the swelling re-accumulated within a day. What is the next most appropriate step in management?

A. Repeat aspiration and apply a compression dressing
B. Prescribe anticholinergic medication
C. Perform sialography to further evaluate the fistula tract
D. Inject botulinum toxin into the parotid gland
E. Excise the skin defect and close it primarily

Q4. A 65-year-old male presents with a painless, slowly enlarging mass in the parotid gland. He has no facial nerve involvement. Fine-needle aspiration cytology (FNAC) suggests features of a malignant salivary gland tumour with basaloid cells arranged in cribriform patterns. What is the most likely diagnosis?

DOI: 10.1201/9781003609308-7

A. Mucoepidermoid carcinoma
B. Adenoid cystic carcinoma
C. Acinic cell carcinoma
D. Adenocarcinoma
E. Malignant mixed tumour

Q5. A 12-year-old undergoes an excisional biopsy of a lump in the lower lip that had been present for an unknown duration. During the procedure, the lesion burst, discharging clear fluid. A small amount of remaining tissue was sent for histological examination, revealing marked cellular atypia. What is the most appropriate next step in management?
A. Observe and monitor for recurrence
B. Repeat excision with wider margins
C. Schedule for radiation therapy to the lower lip
D. Initiate chemotherapy given the cellular atypia
E. Obtain a second opinion from a pathologist for further clarification

Q6. A 50-year-old man presents with recurrent right-sided submandibular swelling and discomfort during meals. Clinical examination suggests mild tenderness in the submandibular region without signs of infection. Imaging confirms a 4 mm radiopaque stone in the distal part of the duct, beyond the mylohyoid muscle, with no evidence of additional stones within the gland. During attempted basket removal with sialendoscopy, it is noted that the stone is firmly lodged in the duct, with slight inflammation in the surrounding tissues. What is the most appropriate next step in management?
A. Observation and re-evaluation after one month
B. Incision of Wharton's duct with sialolithotomy, followed by sialodochoplasty
C. Submandibular gland removal to prevent future recurrence
D. Attempt lithotripsy to fragment the stone for easier removal
E. Intraoperative placement of a Fogarty catheter to dilate the duct and facilitate stone removal

Q7. During a parotidectomy for pleomorphic adenoma in a 35-year-old patient, the capsule of the tumour was inadvertently breached, leading to spillage of tumour cells. The surgeon irrigated the field copiously with isotonic solution. Histopathology confirmed complete removal of the tumour. What is the most appropriate next step in management?
A. Immediate postoperative radiation therapy to the parotid region
B. Observation with regular imaging follow-up
C. Re-operation to achieve complete resection with wide margins
D. Adjuvant radiation therapy after the first recurrence
E. Hypertonic irrigation

Q8. A 40-year-old male undergoes a total parotidectomy for pleomorphic adenoma, resulting in a noticeable divot defect in the preauricular region. Additionally, he has significant facial nerve weakness, leading to incomplete eye closure and asymmetry of the nasolabial fold. What is the most appropriate management plan to address this?

A. Gold weight implantation in the eyelid and dermal fat grafting
B. Cervicofascial rotation flap for the defect and dynamic muscle transfer for facial reanimation
C. ALT free flap to fill the defect and observation for facial nerve function recovery
D. Static sling with ALT fascia lata only, as this will address both volume and reanimation
E. Gold weight implantation alone, as it will improve both eye closure and facial symmetry

Q9. A 72-year-old woman presents with a parotid mass that has grown significantly over the past three months, accompanied by pain and facial nerve weakness. Imaging reveals an irregular mass with heterogeneous enhancement. Fine-needle aspiration shows cells with granular basophilic cytoplasm and round nuclei. What is the most likely diagnosis, and what is the recommended treatment approach?
A. Acinic cell carcinoma; parotidectomy with facial nerve preservation
B. Mucoepidermoid carcinoma; superficial parotidectomy
C. Squamous cell carcinoma metastasis; radical parotidectomy with neck dissection
D. Adenocarcinoma; radiation therapy alone
E. Adenoid cystic carcinoma; parotidectomy with facial nerve preservation

Q10. A 25-year-old patient undergoing excision of a ranula develops brisk arterial bleeding from the floor of the mouth during dissection. Which of the following is true about the vessel most likely responsible for the bleeding?
A. This vessel also supplies the tip of the tongue
B. This vessel also supplies the posterior third of the tongue
C. This vessel also supplies geniohyoid
D. This vessel originates from the facial artery
E. This vessel runs with the superior laryngeal nerve earlier in its course

Q11. An 82-year-old female presents with painful swelling of the right parotid gland. She is currently under investigation due to incidental finding of bilateral hilar lymphadenopathy. A follow-up serum ACE was elevated. She reports low oral intake for the last week. Examination reveals enlarged right preauricular swelling which is tender and firm. She has dry mucous membranes. She is febrile and there is nothing expressible from the duct. Which of the following is the most likely?
A. Heerfordt syndrome
B. Ramsay Hunt syndrome
C. Mumps
D. Bacterial sialadenitis
E. Tuberculosis

Q12: A 55-year-old female had a history of recurrent parotid gland swelling. Sialography six months ago revealed ductal narrowing without stones. She suffers from anxiety and panic disorder for which she is taking SSRIs. She wanted time to consider her options and has returned for review today. She has been symptom free for six months. Her most recent ultrasound (one week old) has shown atrophy of the parotid gland. Which of the following is the best option?

A. Balloon ductal dilation
B. Parotid excision
C. Sialendoscopy with irrigation and intraductual steroids
D. Observation
E. Intraglandal botulinum toxin

Q13. A 20-year-old female presents with a fluctuant, bluish swelling in the floor of the mouth. It has been slowly increasing in size and occasionally causes discomfort during eating. What is the best treatment option?
A. Incision and drainage
B. Sclerotherapy
C. Marsupialisation
D. Sublingual gland excision
E. Observation

Q14. A 60-year-old male presents with a painless mass on the hard palate. Biopsy reveals evidence of malignancy with a solid component and small basaloid epithelial cells. What is the most appropriate management option?
A. Partial excision of the mass with radiotherapy
B. Wide local excision
C. Maxillectomy
D. Curettage and steroid injection
E. Chemoradiotherapy alone

Q15. A 45-year-old female with a history of ranula formation presents for definitive treatment. Workup has shown the ranula plunging into the submandibular triangle. Which of the following provides innervation to the muscle the ranula has herniated through?
A. Lingual nerve
B. Hypoglossal nerve
C. Inferior alveolar nerve
D. Marginal mandibular nerve
E. Glossopharyngeal nerve

Q16. A 58-year-old female undergoes superficial parotidectomy for a pleomorphic adenoma. Postoperatively, she notices sweating in the cheek while eating. You arrange a test to confirm this. What would you expect?
A. Skin in affected area to change reagent red
B. Increased sweating once the reagent is applied to the skin
C. Skin in affected area to change reagent blue/black
D. No colour change
E. Skin in affected area to change reagent brown

Q17. A 63-year-old female presents with a 4 cm pleomorphic adenoma extending into both the superficial and deep lobes of the parotid gland. Which of the following would be the best option?
A. Complete removal of the parotid gland with sacrifice of the facial nerve
B. Removal of the superficial lobe while preserving the deep lobe and the facial nerve

C. Removal of both superficial and deep lobes while preserving the facial nerve
D. Extracapsular dissection of the tumour with limited parotid gland removal
E. Observation

Q18. A 65-year-old male is diagnosed with a high-grade mucoepidermoid carcinoma of the parotid gland invading the facial nerve. What is the most appropriate surgical approach?
A. Total conservative parotidectomy
B. Radical parotidectomy with facial nerve sacrifice
C. Superficial parotidectomy with nerve preservation
D. Extracapsular dissection
E. Endoscopic excision

Q19. A 35-year-old female presents with recurrent submandibular gland swelling due to a 6 mm stone in the proximal Wharton's duct. Which is the most appropriate treatment?
A. Open transoral stone retrieval
B. Endoscopic stone retrieval (sialendoscopy)
C. Submandibular gland excision
D. Shockwave lithotripsy
E. Observation

Q20. A 25-year-old female presents with recurrent submandibular gland swelling and pain during meals. A lower occlusal film shows a 1.5 cm radiopaque lesion medial to the premolars. The patient has COPD and is on apixaban for AF. What is the most appropriate management?
A. Transoral incision at the floor of the mouth
B. Submandibular gland excision
C. Percutaneous ductal approach
D. Endoscopic retrieval via sialendoscopy
E. Buccal mucosal approach

Q21. A 45-year-old male presents with a slow-growing, painless, mobile swelling in the left parotid region. Fine-needle aspiration reveals epithelial and myoepithelial cells within a chondromyxoid stroma. What is the most likely diagnosis?
A. Warthin's tumour
B. Pleomorphic adenoma
C. Adenoid cystic carcinoma
D. Mucoepidermoid carcinoma
E. Basal cell adenoma

Q22. A 45-year-old male presents with a laceration over the cheek in the left preauricular region. What is the best method to confirm parotid duct injury?
A. Inject methylene blue into the duct via a cannula
B. Perform ultrasound of the parotid gland
C. Perform MRI of the face
D. Probe the duct with a lacrimal probe and cannulate
E. Use CT sialography

Q23. A 45-year-old man presents with a complete left facial nerve palsy following a parotidectomy for a high-grade malignancy. He is seeking dynamic reconstructive options to restore facial symmetry and improve his ability to smile. After consultation with the surgical team, he is scheduled for a two-stage, cross-facial nerve graft with muscle transfer. Which of the following statements is correct regarding the management of facial nerve palsy?

A. The sural nerve graft used in cross-facial nerve grafting is typically harvested from the medial aspect of the leg.
B. Masseter muscle transfer involves detaching the muscle from the zygomatic arch and suturing it to the lip for dynamic movement.
C. Electrical stimulation of the grafted muscle postoperatively prevents atrophy during nerve regeneration.
D. Electrical stimulation of the muscle graft is avoided postoperatively to allow for natural regeneration.
E. In the Labbé procedure, gracilis muscle is used for smile restoration.

Q24. A 45-year-old male presents with right-sided facial weakness and difficulty closing his right eye. On examination, he has a loss of taste sensation in the anterior two-thirds of the tongue, and his lacrimal secretion is reduced on the right side. The patient also reports a increased sensitivity to sounds. Based on the anatomy of the facial nerve, which of the following is the most likely site of the lesion?

A. Facial canal after the geniculate ganglion
B. Internal auditory meatus
C. Stylomastoid foramen
D. Intraparotid
E. Pterygopalatine ganglion

Q25. A 55-year-old male, who is a smoker, presents with a painless, slow-growing mass in the right parotid region. On examination, the mass is mobile and well-defined. The patient has no signs of facial nerve involvement. A fine-needle aspiration reveals a mixture of ductal epithelium and lymphoid stroma with occasional germinal centres. What is the most likely diagnosis?

A. Pleomorphic adenoma
B. Warthin's tumour
C. Mucoepidermoid carcinoma
D. Adenoid cystic carcinoma
E. Basal cell adenoma

Q26. A 65-year-old male presents with a firm, painless nodule on his upper lip, which has been gradually enlarging over the past few months. The patient has no significant medical history and is not experiencing any associated symptoms such as pain or facial weakness. On examination, the lesion is well-defined and mobile. Biopsy shows minimal pleomorphism and no invasion. There are basaloid cells in nests with small uniform nuclei and prominent basement membrane-like material surrounding the tumour cell nests. What is the most likely diagnosis?

A. Pleomorphic adenoma
B. Basal cell adenoma
C. Warthin's tumour

D. Mucoepidermoid carcinoma
E. Squamous cell carcinoma

Q27. A 40-year-old female presents with a painful, rapidly enlarging lesion on the hard palate. The lesion initially appeared as a red swelling, which later developed into a crater-like ulcer measuring about 2 cm in diameter. The patient reports a history of smoking and recent dental treatment. There is no significant facial swelling, and the patient denies any systemic symptoms. Biopsy of the lesion shows necrotic tissue with surrounding normal glandular architecture. What is the most likely diagnosis?
A. Oral squamous cell carcinoma
B. Necrotising sialometaplasia
C. Mucoepidermoid carcinoma
D. Atypical odontogenic infection
E. Herpes simplex virus ulceration

ANSWERS AND EXPLANATIONS

Q1. **Sjögren's syndrome diagnosis**

Answer: D. Lower labial gland biopsy

Explanation: This patient has systemic lupus erythematosus and symptoms consistent with secondary Sjögren's syndrome, supported by subjective symptoms (dry mouth and eyes) and positive autoantibodies (anti-Ro/SS-A, anti-La/SS-B). Secondary Sjögren's syndrome diagnosis requires one subjective and two objective features, and a lower labial gland biopsy showing focal lymphocytic infiltration is a definitive objective test that would support the diagnosis. Although salivary scintigraphy and Schirmer test could offer additional information, the biopsy provides direct histopathological confirmation, making it the most useful next test in this context.

Q2. **Complications of Sjögren's syndrome**

Answer: D. Open parotid biopsy of the lesion

Explanation: Unilateral parotid gland enlargement in a patient with primary Sjögren's syndrome, especially in the presence of systemic symptoms (fever, fatigue, weight loss) and a single hypoechoic lesion, is concerning for MALT lymphoma. While fine-needle aspiration could provide preliminary information, an open biopsy is preferred in this context to obtain sufficient tissue for a definitive histopathological diagnosis. High-dose corticosteroids would not address a potential malignancy, and pilocarpine would only relieve symptoms temporarily without addressing the underlying cause.

Q3. **Sialocele management**

Answer: B. Prescribe anticholinergic medication

Explanation: This patient's presentation suggests a postoperative sialocele with transformation into a salivary fistula, as evidenced by the clear fluid drainage and elevated amylase levels. Although aspiration with compression is often the first-line treatment for a sialocele, re-accumulation after multiple aspirations suggests further treatment is required. Botulinum toxin is an option in refractory cases but would not be the immediate next step in this case. Anticholinergics may help reduce salivary output.

Q4. **Adenoid cystic carcinoma**

Answer: B. Adenoid cystic carcinoma

Explanation: The description of basaloid cells arranged in cribriform patterns on FNAC is characteristic of adenoid cystic carcinoma, a malignant tumour commonly found in the parotid and other salivary glands. This tumour is well-known for its tendency toward perineural invasion, even in the absence of facial nerve symptoms at presentation. Mucoepidermoid carcinoma is the most common malignant tumour in the parotid. Acinic cell carcinoma predominantly occurs in the parotid and histological features are of serous acinar differentiation and basophilic cytoplasmic granules. Adenocarcinoma and malignant mixed tumours can exhibit aggressive behaviour but do not display the unique cribriform architecture and perineural invasion typical of adenoid cystic carcinoma.

Q5. **Interpreting histological findings**

Answer: B. Repeat excision with wider margins

Explanation: The histology indicating marked cellular atypia suggests that the lesion may be malignant or pre-malignant. Although the lesion ruptured and discharged clear fluid, which might suggest a benign lesion such as a mucocele, the presence of cellular atypia raises suspicion for a malignant or dysplastic process that warrants a more definitive treatment. Repeat excision with wider margins is the most appropriate course to ensure complete removal of any residual atypical or malignant tissue. Observation would be inappropriate given the histological findings, and radiation therapy or chemotherapy would not be indicated without a confirmed diagnosis of malignancy. A second pathological review could be helpful, but the priority is to ensure adequate excision with clear margins.

Q6. **Sialolith management**

Answer: B. Incision of Wharton's duct with sialolithotomy, followed by sialodochoplasty

Explanation: This patient has a distal stone in Wharton's duct beyond the mylohyoid muscle, which makes it accessible for direct ductal incision (sialolithotomy) with sialodochoplasty. Given the stone's location and size, this approach is preferable to avoid more invasive gland removal and to preserve salivary function. Observation is not appropriate, as the patient has recurrent symptoms and a clearly defined obstructive stone. Submandibular gland removal is generally reserved for stones located at the proximal end or within the gland itself, especially when they are difficult to access directly. Lithotripsy is typically used for larger, more proximal stones rather than small, distal ones. Although a Fogarty catheter can be useful in displacing a mobile stone, this stone is noted to be firmly lodged, so direct incision and stone extraction are necessary.

Q7. **Management of tumour spillage**

Answer: B. Observation with regular imaging follow-up

Explanation: The management of pleomorphic adenoma after intraoperative tumour spillage is controversial. While tumour spillage can theoretically increase recurrence risk, it does not guarantee recurrence. Current evidence suggests that immediate postoperative radiation therapy (RT) is not routinely recommended due to the low recurrence rate after the first surgery and potential complications of RT, such as xerostomia and neural dysfunction. Observation with regular imaging is often preferred, especially in young patients, allowing for early detection of recurrence if it occurs. Re-operation is generally not indicated unless there is clear evidence of residual tumour. Adjuvant RT may be considered only after documented recurrence, especially in younger patients, due to the increased risk of nerve damage in subsequent surgeries. Hypertonic irrigation lacks evidence for effectiveness in reducing recurrence risk compared to isotonic solution.

Q8. **Facial nerve weakness post-parotidectomy**

Answer: A. Gold weight implantation in the eyelid and dermal fat grafting

Explanation: Following total parotidectomy, facial contour defects and facial nerve dysfunction are common. A preauricular divot defect can be managed effectively with autologous fat grafting or dermal fat grafting to restore volume. Facial nerve weakness, particularly lagophthalmos, can be addressed with gold weight implantation in the upper eyelid to improve eyelid closure and prevent exposure keratopathy. Both of these are simple interventions with little morbidity. Static facial suspension techniques may be considered later on for nasolabial fold asymmetry if dynamic reanimation is not possible. Immediate nerve grafting is usually only feasible in cases of intraoperative nerve injury rather than delayed paralysis. While free flap reconstruction with masseteric nerve transfer is an option for dynamic reanimation, it is typically reserved for cases with long-standing paralysis. RT has no role in managing these post-surgical deficits.

Q9. **Acinic cell carcinoma**

Answer: A. Acinic cell carcinoma; parotidectomy with facial nerve preservation

Explanation: The FNAC findings of basophilic granular cytoplasm and round nuclei suggest acinic cell carcinoma, which is a malignant tumour of the parotid gland but generally has a more favourable prognosis than other malignancies. Although this patient presents with facial nerve weakness, indicating possible nerve involvement, the standard treatment approach for acinic cell carcinoma typically includes parotidectomy with attempts to preserve the facial nerve if feasible. Weakness may be secondary to compression rather than invasion. Mucoepidermoid carcinoma and adenoid cystic carcinoma could also cause facial nerve involvement, but their cytological appearances differ from that of acinic cell carcinoma. Radiation therapy (RT) alone is not the primary treatment for salivary gland malignancies.

Q10. **Anatomy of the floor of mouth**

Answer: C. This vessel also supplies geniohyoid

Explanation: The sublingual artery, a branch of the lingual artery, is the most likely source of bleeding during ranula excision. It supplies the floor of the mouth, the sublingual gland, and muscles including geniohyoid. The other branches of the lignual artery are the dorsal lingual artery supplying the posterior third and the deep lingual artery supplying the tip of the tongue. The superior laryngeal nerve runs with the superior thyroid artery in the neck.

Q11. **Bacterial sialadenitis**

Answer: D. Bacterial sialadenitis

Explanation: Although the stem is distracting as it suggests a new diagnosis of Sarcoidosis, the clinical picture is classic for parotitis given the unilateral swelling in the context of a dehydrated, febrile elderly patient. There is no mention of facial palsy excluding Heerfordt and Ramsay Hunt. The most common bacterial causes of sialadenitis are Staphylococcus aureus, streptococci, and Haemophilus influenzae.

Q12. **Salivary duct stenosis**

Answer: D. Observation

Explanation: Although minimally invasive procedures have vastly improved management of salivary strictures, they are not without risk. Stenoses associated with recognisable atrophy of the gland or asymptomatic stenoses do not require intervention and can be monitored (12).

Q13. **Ranula management**

Answer: D. Sublingual gland excision

Explanation: Definitive treatment of ranulas involves excision of the sublingual gland to prevent recurrence. Marsupialisation alone has a high recurrence rate.

Q14. **Adenoid cystic carcinoma**

Answer: B. Wide local excision

Explanation: Adenoid cystic carcinoma (ACC) is a malignant salivary gland tumour known for its slow but relentless progression, high risk of perineural invasion, and tendency for local recurrence. Wide local excision is the treatment of choice to achieve clear margins and reduce the risk of recurrence. Maxillectomy may be required for extensive lesions involving the bony palate, but smaller tumours can often be managed with wide local excision alone. Radiotherapy may be considered as an adjuvant treatment in cases with positive margins or perineural invasion, but chemoradiotherapy alone is insufficient for definitive management. Curettage and steroid injection have no role in treating malignant salivary gland tumours. Given ACC's aggressive nature and high recurrence potential, long-term follow-up is essential.

Q15. **Anatomy of the floor of the mouth**

Answer: C. Inferior alveolar nerve

Explanation: Ranulas herniate through mylohyoid when plunging into the neck. The nerve to mylohyoid, which also innervates the anterior belly of digastric, is a branch off the inferior alveolar nerve.

Q16. **Frey's syndrome**

Answer: C. Skin in affected area to change reagent blue/black

Explanation: Frey's syndrome occurs due to aberrant regeneration of parasympathetic fibres to sweat glands after parotidectomy. The ipsilateral face is painted with iodine and allowed to dry. Starch powder is dusted onto the face. The patient is given a sialogogue. Dark blue/black staining reveals the affected area.

Q17. **Total parotidectomy**

Answer: C. Removal of both superficial and deep lobes while preserving the facial nerve

Explanation: Total conservative parotidectomy involves removal of both the superficial and deep lobes of the parotid gland while preserving the facial nerve. It is typically indicated for large benign tumours involving both lobes.

Q18. **Radical parotidectomy**

Answer: B. Radical parotidectomy with facial nerve sacrifice

Explanation: Radical parotidectomy involves removal of the entire parotid, gland along with the facial nerve and any involved surrounding structures. It is indicated for malignant tumours with nerve invasion.

Q19. **Sialendoscopy**

Answer: B. Endoscopic stone retrieval (sialendoscopy)

Explanation: Sialendoscopy is a minimally invasive approach to manage salivary stones and strictures, avoiding gland excision and reducing morbidity. For a 6 mm stone in the proximal Wharton's duct, endoscopic retrieval is preferred, as it provides direct visualisation and allows for precise stone removal. This approach also preserves gland function and minimises the risks associated with open surgery or gland excision (13).

Q20. **Sialolith management**

Answer: A. Transoral incision at the floor of the mouth

Explanation: Large stones located near the opening of Wharton's duct are typically removed via a transoral incision at the floor of the mouth. Different techniques are described to minimise risk of sialolith displacement, iatrogenic injury to lingual nerve and postoperative duct stenosis.

Q21. **Pleomorphic adenoma**

Answer: B. Pleomorphic adenoma

Explanation: Pleomorphic adenoma is the most common benign salivary gland tumour. It is characterised histologically by a mixture of epithelial and myoepithelial cells in a chondromyxoid stroma. Warthin's tumour has a lymphoid stroma and is less common.

Q22. **Parotid duct injury**

Answer: D. Probe the duct with a lacrimal probe and cannulate

Explanation: An easy way to diagnose the presence of injury to the parotid gland is by palpating and massaging the gland to express saliva into the field. If there is injury to the ductal structures, saliva will be seen pooling in the wound. To confirm the presence of ductal injury, cannulate the duct from its distal oral opening with a paediatric intravenous catheter after dilating it with a lacrimal probe and inject saline or methylene blue. If the injected liquid does not appear in the wound, the ductal system is intact. Methylene blue should be injected with caution because it can discolour the surgical field *and* make identification of the facial nerve very difficult. Magnetic resonance imaging and computed tomography are not useful in assessing parotid trauma. Sialography can confirm ductal system integrity but may be difficult to access in the acute setting (14).

Q23. **Facial nerve weakness post-parotidectomy**

Answer: C. Electrical stimulation of the grafted muscle postoperatively prevents atrophy during nerve regeneration.

Explanation: Dynamic reconstruction of facial nerve palsy aims to restore movement and symmetry. Cross-facial nerve grafting with muscle transfer is a well-established technique for achieving dynamic reanimation. Electrical stimulation of the grafted muscle postoperatively is crucial to prevent atrophy and maintain muscle tone while waiting for nerve regeneration, which typically starts 9–15 months after surgery. The sural nerve is harvested from the posterior-lateral aspect of the leg, not the medial aspect (medially is the saphenous nerve). The Labbé procedure (lengthening temporalis myoplasty) uses the temporalis muscle for smile restoration, not gracilis. Masseter muscle transfer involves its transposition but does not involve detachment from the zygomatic arch.

Q24. **Facial nerve anatomy**

Answer: B. Internal auditory meatus

Explanation: The patient's symptoms—right-sided facial weakness, loss of taste sensation in the anterior two-thirds of the tongue, reduced lacrimal secretion, and hyperacusis—are indicative of a lesion affecting the facial nerve before it branches out to the extratemporal region. The facial nerve exits the brainstem at the pons; travels through the internal auditory meatus, along with the vestibulocochlear nerve (CN VIII); and enters the facial canal within the temporal bone. A lesion at the internal auditory meatus would affect both the motor and sensory components of the facial nerve, leading to facial paralysis (due to the motor nucleus), loss of taste (due to the chorda tympani), reduced lacrimation (due to the greater petrosal nerve), and potential hearing issues (due to the stapedius nerve). This corresponds with the clinical presentation in the question. Lesions at other locations such as the geniculate ganglion involve specific branches of the facial nerve but would not explain the combination of symptoms seen here. The pterygopalatine ganglion is not involved in the motor function or taste sensation and would not account for the facial weakness or other findings.

Q25. **Warthin's tumour**

Answer: B. Warthin's tumour

Explanation: Warthin's tumour (also known as papillary cystadenoma lymphomatosum) is the second most common benign tumour of the parotid gland. It is strongly associated with smoking, which is a key factor in this patient's history. The tumour is typically characterised by a benign proliferation of entrapped salivary gland cells in lymphoid elements. Histologically, it usually shows ductal epithelium and lymphoid stroma, and may contain germinal centres, as noted in the fine-needle aspiration report. Warthin's tumours are often mobile and well-defined on examination, and they rarely involve the facial nerve.

Q26. **Basal cell adenoma**

Answer: B. Basal cell adenoma

Explanation: Basal cell adenoma is a rare benign tumour that typically presents as small, painless nodules. While it is most commonly found in the parotid gland (about 70% of cases), it can also present in the upper lip, as seen in this patient (20% of cases). The lesion is usually firm, well-defined, and mobile, with a slow and painless growth pattern. Basal cell adenoma is most commonly seen in individuals aged 60–70. Although benign, basal cell adenoma has the potential to transform into basal cell adenocarcinoma, a malignant form, in rare cases.

Q27. **Necrotising sialometaplasia**

Answer: B. Necrotising sialometaplasia

Explanation: Necrotising sialometaplasia (NSM) is a benign condition of the salivary glands, most commonly affecting the hard palate, although other sites such as the buccal mucosa and floor of mouth can also be involved. It typically presents with an acute onset of erythematous swelling followed by the development of a crater-like ulcer, measuring 1–3 cm in diameter. Pain and rapid progression are common, and the lesion usually heals within 3–12 weeks. The condition is strongly associated with smoking, trauma (including dental procedures), and other factors, such as alcohol or drug use. While it has a characteristic clinical course, the aggressive appearance of the lesion can mimic malignancy, which is why biopsy is often performed to rule out neoplastic causes.

7 Craniofacial Deformity and Cleft

QUESTIONS

Q1. A 17-year-old patient presents with progressive facial asymmetry and chin deviation towards the left side. Examination reveals unilateral horizontal enlargement of the right mandible with no transverse canting of the occlusal plane. Imaging confirms active condylar growth on the affected side. What is the most appropriate next step in management?

A. Orthognathic surgery to correct the mandibular asymmetry
B. Orthodontic alignment and occlusal adjustments
C. Condylectomy of the affected side
D. Genioplasty to mask the asymmetry
E. Observation until growth has completely stopped

Q2. A 3-month-old is found to have a divergent gaze, and the left side of the face shows an inability to frown, smile, or close the eye. The parents think this has been present since birth. What is the most likely diagnosis?

A. Möbius syndrome
B. Congenital ptosis
C. Bell's palsy
D. Goldenhar syndrome
E. Treacher-Collins syndrome

Q3. During mandibular distraction osteogenesis, which of the following phases involves active elongation of the bone?

A. Latency phase
B. Consolidation phase
C. Remodelling phase
D. Distraction phase
E. Corticotomy

Q4. A 20-year-old male presents with facial asymmetry and ipsilateral enlargement of the right mandible, including the condyle and ramus. Which feature best differentiates hemimandibular hyperplasia from hemimandibular elongation?

A. Open bite
B. Increased vertical growth of the ramus
C. Lateral displacement of the chin to ipsilateral side
D. Ipsilateral crossbite
E. Midline shift to contralateral side

Q5. A 30-year-old patient presents with a history of facial asymmetry and chin deviation to the left. Examination reveals a three-dimensional enlargement of the right

DOI: 10.1201/9781003609308-8

mandible with transverse canting of the occlusal plane and supraeruption of the maxillary molars on the affected side. Imaging confirms that condylar growth has stopped. What is the most appropriate management option?
A. Orthodontics and condylectomy of the affected side
B. Orthodontics combined with bilateral sagittal split osteotomy (BSSO) and genioplasty
C. Orthodontics combined with Le Fort 1 osteotomy, BSSO, and genioplasty
D. Orthodontics and genioplasty
E. Orthodontics and reduction of the inferior border of the mandible on the affected side

Q6. A 15-year-old patient presents with a bluish, compressible swelling on the left cheek that blanches on pressure and becomes more prominent when lying down or straining. The lesion has been present since birth but has grown in size during adolescence. What is the most appropriate initial treatment option?
A. Pulsed dye laser therapy
B. Complete surgical excision
C. Sclerotherapy with sclerosant agents
D. Conventional angiography with embolisation
E. Observation and reassurance

Q7. What is the main reason cleft palate repair is typically performed at around 12 months of age according to most surgical protocols?
A. To support speech and language development
B. The size of the cleft defect
C. The likelihood of velopharyngeal insufficiency
D. The patient's overall health and nutritional condition
E. The presence of associated syndromes

Q8. Which surgical approach is most effective in restoring lip symmetry and functional movement during unilateral cleft lip repair?
A. Repositioning of the levator labii superioris
B. Realignment of the orbicularis oris
C. Augmentation of the nasal base
D. Using Z-plasty to lengthen the columella
E. Refining the Cupid's bow

Q9. During bilateral cleft lip repair, what is the primary purpose of using the vomer flap in the early stages of surgical correction?
A. To prevent disturbances in maxillary growth
B. To support the structure of the nasal septum
C. To establish continuity of the nasal floor
D. To avoid fistula formation between the oral and nasal cavities
E. To realign the orbicularis oris at the midline

Q10. A 3-year-old child with hemifacial microsomia presents with significant mandibular hypoplasia, resulting in difficulty breathing and feeding. Which of the following is the most appropriate initial management step?
A. Insertion of Hickman line for long-term total parenteral nutrition (TPN)

B. Mandibular lengthening using distraction osteogenesis
C. Placement of a tracheostomy and nasogastric tube
D. Conventional orthognathic surgery
E. Malar augmentation

Q11. A 17-year-old patient presents with a mandibular arteriovenous malformation (AVM) causing intermittent bleeding and significant facial swelling. Imaging confirms a high-flow lesion with a central nidus involving the mandibular bone. What is the most appropriate initial management?
A. Conservative monitoring
B. Surgical resection with mandibular reconstruction
C. Embolisation followed by surgical resection
D. Radiation therapy
E. Simple embolisation

Q12. Why is it important to stage cleft lip and palate repair, beginning with lip repair followed by hard and soft palate repairs?
A. To reduce the risk of maxillary growth restriction
B. To prevent velopharyngeal insufficiency as speech develops
C. To improve the child's nutritional status over time
D. To minimise the likelihood of postoperative fistula formation
E. To enhance the function of the velopharyngeal mechanism

Q13. What is the optimal stage of dental development for secondary alveolar bone grafting in cleft palate patients to achieve the best outcomes?
A. Before the first molar erupts
B. After the central incisors have erupted
C. When the permanent canine's root development is between 1/2 and 2/3 complete
D. Once the permanent lateral incisor is fully erupted
E. After the permanent canine has erupted

Q14. A 2-year-old child with coronal craniosynostosis presents with significant forehead retrusion, orbital dystopia, and mild intracranial hypertension. Which of the following surgical approaches best addresses the functional and aesthetic concerns associated with this condition?
A. Fronto-orbital remodelling with advancement and calvarial reshaping
B. Posterior vault distraction osteogenesis followed by delayed orbital correction
C. Isolated orbital rim advancement with titanium implants
D. Total cranial vault reconstruction with reshaping of the frontal bone
E. Endoscopic cranial suturectomy with postoperative helmet therapy

Q15. A 10-month-old infant is diagnosed with metopic craniosynostosis, leading to a trigonocephalic deformity. The child is exhibiting signs of increased intracranial pressure and developmental delay. What is the most appropriate management strategy?
A. Delayed surgical correction until 18 months to allow further cranial growth
B. Endoscopic strip craniectomy followed by helmet therapy
C. Total cranial vault remodelling surgery

D. Observation with regular monitoring of developmental milestones
E. Cranial distraction osteogenesis with gradual expansion

Q16. A newborn is noted to have a midline facial defect extending from the upper lip through the nose and into the forehead, associated with hypotelorism and a single central incisor. Which classification system would most accurately describe this cleft?
A. Veau classification
B. Kernahan and Stark classification
C. Tessier classification
D. American Cleft Palate Association classification
E. Harkins and Converse classification

Q17. A 6-month-old infant with a bilateral Tessier 4 craniofacial cleft presents for surgical repair. The cleft involves the upper lip, maxilla, and extends to the lower eyelid, causing significant coloboma and midface asymmetry. Which surgical approach would best address both the functional and aesthetic deformities in this case?
A. Primary repair of the soft tissue components only, followed by delayed skeletal repair
B. Simultaneous repair of the soft tissue cleft and midface advancement using distraction osteogenesis
C. Staged soft tissue repair followed by Le Fort I osteotomy in adolescence
D. Comprehensive soft tissue repair combined with midface skeletal repositioning using a frontofacial monobloc advancement
E. Isolated orbital floor reconstruction with skin grafting for coloboma correction

Q18. A 13-year-old patient with hemifacial microsomia presents for evaluation of facial asymmetry. Examination reveals mild hypoplasia of the mandible, maxillary canting, and a moderate pinna abnormality. Which of the following is the most appropriate next step in management?
A. Bone-anchored hearing aid placement
B. Le Fort I osteotomy and active orthodontics
C. Autologous costochondral graft for pinna reconstruction
D. Fat transfer for soft tissue augmentation
E. Observation until skeletal growth is complete

Q19. A 12-year-old male presents with a flat, underdeveloped midface, a short nose, and a flat nasal bridge. Examination reveals midfacial hypoplasia, a prominent lower jaw, and a reverse overjet. Imaging shows an underdeveloped premaxilla and absence of the anterior nasal spine. Which of the following is also likely to be present?
A. Multiple basal cell carcinomas and keratocystic odontogenic tumours
B. Hypocalcaemia and a history of congenital heart defects
C. Fusion of the first and second cervical vertebrae
D. Craniosynostosis with shallow orbits and hypertelorism
E. Oral fibrous papules and intestinal hamartomatous polyps

Q20. A 15-year-old male presents with significant facial asymmetry and hypertelorism following repair of a Tessier 3 craniofacial cleft during early childhood. Examination reveals orbital dystopia, including downward displacement of the right orbit with vertical diplopia. What is the most appropriate surgical approach to address this condition?

A. Orbital roof reconstruction using titanium mesh
B. Distraction osteogenesis of the zygomatic complex
C. Monobloc advancement with midface and orbital repositioning
D. Osteotomy and repositioning of the orbital floor with soft tissue adjustment
E. Endoscopic medial wall repositioning with alloplastic graft placement

Q21. A 2-month-old infant presents with a midline facial cleft. Embryologically, failure of which of the following processes is most likely responsible for this presentation?

A. Fusion of the medial nasal and maxillary prominences
B. Fusion of the lateral nasal and maxillary prominences
C. Formation of the frontal bone from the neural crest
D. Fusion of the mandibular prominences
E. Closure of the anterior neuropore

Q22. A 6-year-old boy presents with mandibular hypoplasia, auricular deformity, and an epibulbar dermoid. Genetic testing identifies a de novo mutation. Which of the following is most commonly associated with this condition?

A. Mutations in the TCOF1 gene
B. Chromosome 22q11.2 deletion
C. Mutations in the FGFR2 gene
D. Pathogenic variant in the EYA1 gene
E. Mutations in the SALL4 gene

Q23. A 3-month-old presents with a midline scalp defect containing neural tissue. This condition is most likely caused by failure of which of the following embryologic processes?

A. Neural crest migration into the calvarium
B. Primary neurulation
C. Fusion of the secondary palate
D. Somite differentiation into sclerotomes
E. Closure of the posterior neuropore

Q24. A 14-year-old boy presents with café-au-lait macules, axillary freckling, and a large plexiform neurofibroma on the face. Which of the following genetic abnormalities is most likely responsible for this presentation?

A. Mutation in the NF1 gene on chromosome 17
B. Mutation in the NF2 gene on chromosome 22
C. Deletion of the PTEN gene
D. Mutation in the TP53 gene
E. Chromosome 22q11 deletion

Q25. A 14-year-old girl presents with occipital headaches, neck pain, and progressive ataxia. MRI reveals her cerebellar tonsils extending 8 mm below the foramen magnum. Which of the following is the most likely primary pathological mechanism underlying her condition?

A. Excessive production of cerebrospinal fluid (CSF)
B. Obstruction of CSF flow
C. Premature fusion of the cranial sutures
D. Enlargement of the foramen magnum
E. Cerebral cortical atrophy

Q26. A 15-year-old patient with a repaired unilateral cleft lip and palate presents for secondary cleft rhinoplasty. What is the primary goal of this procedure?

A. Widening the nasal base
B. Correcting nasal asymmetry and septal deviation
C. Lengthening the nasal tip projection
D. Reducing the nostril size
E. Improving nasal airflow without addressing aesthetic concerns

Q27. An 11-year-old patient who underwent alveolar bone grafting for a unilateral cleft lip and palate is reviewed postoperatively. Radiographic assessment reveals that the bone level in the interdental septum on the graft side is at 80% of the height of the contralateral side. How should this outcome be classified?

A. Bergland Grade I
B. Bergland Grade II
C. Chelsea Category F
D. Kindelan Grade 3
E. Kindelan Grade 4

Q28. A 7-year-old patient with a history of cleft palate repair presents with hypernasality and inadequate lateral wall movement. Which of the following best describes the Orticochea pharyngoplasty procedure?

A. Creation of a superiorly based pharyngeal flap
B. Use of buccal fat pad for defect closure
C. Bilateral posterior pharyngeal flaps to narrow the velopharyngeal gap
D. Lengthening of the soft palate with Z-plasty
E. Palatal muscle retro-positioning

Q29. A 3-year-old child presents with persistent velopharyngeal insufficiency (VPI) after cleft palate repair. Which of the following surgical approaches is most appropriate for addressing a small velopharyngeal gap (<9 mm)?

A. Pharyngeal flap
B. Buccal fat pad flap
C. Furlow double-opposing Z-plasty
D. Sphincter pharyngoplasty
E. Primary palatoplasty

Q30. A 10-year-old child with a history of cleft palate repair presents with a persistent palatal fistula and associated oronasal communication. Orthopantogram reveals the permanent canine's root is 75% developed. What is the next best step in managing this patient?

A. Immediate closure of the fistula with soft tissue repair
B. Secondary alveolar bone graft
C. Delayed bone grafting after complete eruption of permanent canine
D. Speech therapy
E. Use of obturator prosthesis

Q31. A 1-year-old child presents with a cleft palate involving the uvula, soft palate, and hard palate, extending to the alveolus. The child has hypernasal speech and difficulty with feeding. What is the most appropriate management at this stage?
A. Immediate closure of the fistula with soft tissue repair
B. Alveolar bone graft to support maxillary growth
C. Palatoplasty to repair the cleft and improve speech
D. Placement of a prosthetic obturator until adolescence
E. Velopharyngeal augmentation surgery

Q32. A 5-year-old child presents with velopharyngeal insufficiency, recurrent otitis media, and a history of tetralogy of Fallot repair. On examination, the child has a long face, small palpebral fissures, and hypoplastic alae nasi. Which of the following is the most likely additional finding in this condition?
A. Hypercalcaemia due to parathyroid hyperplasia
B. Thymic hypoplasia leading to immunodeficiency
C. Bilateral microtia and conductive hearing loss
D. Macroglossia with hypothyroidism
E. Retinal detachment due to connective tissue disorder

Q33. A newborn is observed to have micrognathia, glossoptosis, and airway obstruction requiring prone positioning for feeding. What is the most appropriate next step in management?
A. Perform mandibular distraction osteogenesis
B. Place a nasopharyngeal airway
C. Insert a gastrostomy tube
D. Perform tracheostomy
E. Refer for genetic testing for Stickler syndrome

Q34. A 10-year-old boy with a history of cleft palate repair presents with progressive hearing loss, joint hypermobility, and myopia. Examination reveals a flattened midface and a history of retinal detachment in the family. What is the most likely underlying genetic abnormality in this condition?
A. Mutation in the FGFR2 gene
B. Mutation in the COL2A1 gene
C. Deletion of the 22q11.2 region
D. Mutation in the TP63 gene
E. Mutation in the TBX1 gene

Q35. A 7-year-old child with a repaired cleft palate presents with hypernasal speech and nasal air emission during consonant production. What is the most likely anatomical cause of these findings?

A. Palatal fistula
B. Overcorrection of the palate
C. Posterior pharyngeal wall defect
D. Velopharyngeal insufficiency
E. Nasal septal deviation

Q36. A 16-year-old patient with a history of cleft palate repair complains of persistent nasal regurgitation and difficulty swallowing. Examination shows a notched posterior hard palate. What is the most likely complication?
A. Adhesion of soft palate to pharyngeal wall
B. Palatal scar hypertrophy
C. Oronasal fistula
D. Overlengthening of the soft palate
E. Velopharyngeal dysfunction

Q37. A 4-year-old child with a history of cleft palate repair is evaluated for chronic middle ear infections and hearing loss. Which is the best explanation of this complication?
A. Dysfunction of the tensor veli palatini muscle
B. Recurrent upper respiratory tract infections
C. Scarring of the eustachian tube
D. Narrowing of the pharyngeal airway
E. Immature immune system

Q38. A 1-month-old infant with a complete cleft palate and lip is evaluated for feeding difficulties and poor weight gain. What is the primary mechanism causing feeding difficulty in such cases?
A. Decreased tongue strength limiting effective latch
B. Reduced intraoral pressure caused by incomplete lip seal
C. Poor coordination of swallowing due to velopharyngeal incompetence
D. Inability to generate suction due to palatal defect
E. Ineffective peristalsis secondary to nasal regurgitation

Q39. A 12-year-old child with a repaired cleft palate presents with hypernasality during speech. Nasopharyngoscopy reveals a circular velopharyngeal closure pattern with significant lateral wall motion but minimal palatal movement. Which surgical procedure is most appropriate for this patient?
A. Pharyngeal flap surgery
B. Sphincter pharyngoplasty
C. Furlow palatoplasty
D. Posterior pharyngeal wall augmentation
E. Speech therapy

Q40. A 2-day-old newborn presents with a bilateral cleft lip and palate. Which genetic syndrome is most likely associated with this presentation?
A. Pierre Robin sequence
B. Van der Woude syndrome
C. Treacher-Collins syndrome
D. Apert syndrome
E. Crouzon syndrome

Q41. A 6-month-old infant with a complete unilateral cleft lip and palate is scheduled for surgical repair. According to standard repair protocols, which of the following should be performed first?

A. Lip adhesion procedure
B. Hard palate repair
C. Soft palate repair
D. Definitive lip repair
E. Pharyngoplasty

Q42. A 3-month-old infant with a unilateral cleft lip is evaluated prior to surgical repair. The embryological failure responsible for this anomaly most likely involves which of the following processes?

A. Failure of mandibular and maxillary processes to merge
B. Failure of lateral nasal and medial nasal processes to merge
C. Failure of maxillary and medial nasal processes to merge
D. Failure of primary and secondary palates to merge
E. Failure of palatal shelves to elevate

Q43. A 4-month-old baby is brought to the clinic by their parents with concerns about an abnormal head shape. The parents noticed flattening of the back of the baby's head on the right side, which developed over the last few months. Examination reveals the following:

- Flattening of the right posterior skull
- Forward displacement of the right ear
- Bossing of the right frontal area and left parietal area

Which of the following statements is **true**?

A. Surgical correction is the treatment of choice.
B. The condition is associated with premature fusion of the lambdoid suture.
C. Helmet therapy is highly effective and recommended for all cases.
D. Tummy time and positional changes are the first-line management.
E. The condition will likely lead to facial and TMJ abnormalities if untreated.

Q44. An 11-year-old male who recently immigrated is brought to the clinic with an untreated unilateral cleft lip on the left side. On examination, you note characteristic anatomical abnormalities associated with the condition. Which of the following statements is **correct**?

A. The nasal tip is deflected to the left side and flattened.
B. The philtral column will be lengthened on the left side.
C. Cupid's bow is rotated towards the right side.
D. Distortions or substitutions of plosives such as "p" and "b" may occur.
E. The nasal septum is typically unaffected by this condition.

Q45. A 6-month-old infant with a wide unilateral cleft lip is being considered for surgical repair using the Tennison-Randall approach. Which of the following statements most accurately describes the key feature of this technique?

A. The Z-plasty is performed on the noncleft side to restore the Cupid's bow symmetry.

B. A triangular flap based laterally is used to fill the deficiency in lip height, with a back-cut extending from the cleft Cupid's bow peak toward the centre of the philtrum.
C. The technique uses a straight-line closure along the cleft lip to restore symmetry.
D. The triangular flap is placed 4 mm above the vermillion to optimise the definition of the white roll on the repaired side.
E. The technique is particularly useful for narrow clefts with minimal vertical lip deficiency.

Q46. A 3-month-old infant with a unilateral cleft lip is being considered for surgical repair using the Millard approach. Which of the following statements best describes the key feature of this technique?
A. The technique relies on a single, straight-line incision that rotates the medial lip segment and advances the lateral lip segment to close the cleft.
B. A curvilinear incision extends from the Cupid's bow peak toward the non-cleft philtral column, allowing for rotation and advancement to correct the cleft deformity.
C. The advancement flap is always designed to include a portion of the nasal floor for correction of the alar flare and narrowing of the nostril floor.
D. The Mohler modification of Millard's repair utilises the columella to lengthen the lip, with a rotation incision that involves the columella but does not involve the philtrum.
E. The rotation-advancement incision is limited to the medial side of the cleft, with no incision made on the lateral lip to avoid disrupting the nasal base.

ANSWERS AND EXPLANATIONS

Q1. **Hemimandibular elongation**

Answer: C. Condylectomy of the affected side

Explanation: The patient presents with features consistent with hemimandibular elongation, including horizontal enlargement of one side of the mandible and chin deviation towards the opposite side, with no transverse canting of the occlusal plane. Given the confirmed active condylar growth, a condylectomy (removal of the superior aspect of the condyle) is indicated to halt further asymmetric growth. Orthognathic surgery and orthodontic adjustments are typically reserved for patients whose growth has ceased, while genioplasty is used to mask asymmetry without correcting the underlying skeletal issue. Observation alone may lead to worsening asymmetry due to continued growth.

Q2. **Möbius syndrome**

Answer: A. Möbius syndrome

Explanation: Möbius syndrome is a rare, non-progressive congenital neurological disorder primarily marked by underdevelopment of the facial nerve (cranial nerve VII) and the abducens nerve (cranial nerve VI).

Q3. **Distraction osteogenesis**

Answer: D. Distraction phase

Explanation: The phases of distraction osteogenesis are as follows:

Corticotomy: Division of the cortical bone to enable distraction.

Latency: Time between osteotomy and initiation of distraction. 3–7 days depending on clinical circumstances.

Distraction:

- Active separation of bone ends.
- Recommended rate: **1 mm/day** (or **1.5 mm/day** in children under 6 to avoid premature consolidation).
- Rhythm: **0.5 mm twice daily** is more effective than a single 1 mm increment.

Consolidation: The callus matures and ossifies.

Q4. **Obwegeser and Makek classification of condylar hyperplasia (1986)**

Answer: A. Open bite

Explanation: Obwegeser and Makek Classification of Condylar Hyperplasia (1986) (15)

Type 1: Hemimandibular Elongation

- **Clinical Findings**:
  - Chin deviation towards the contralateral side
  - Midline shift towards the contralateral side
  - Posterior crossbite on the contralateral side

- **Histological Findings**:
  - Excessive growth in the horizontal vector
  - Enlarged ramus, normal condyle

Type 2: Hemimandibular Hyperplasia

- **Clinical Findings**:
  - Sloping rima oris with minimal chin deviation
  - Supraeruption of maxillary molars on the affected side
  - Open bite
  - Midline shift (minimal to none)

- **Histological Findings**:
  - Excessive growth in the vertical vector
  - Excessive growth in the condylar head

Type 3: Combination of Both

- **Clinical Findings**:
  - Chin deviation towards the contralateral side
  - Possible open bite
  - Sloping rima oris with possible chin deviation

- **Histological Findings**:
  - Combination of excessive growth in both vectors

Q5. **Hemimandibular hyperplasia**

Answer: C. Orthodontics combined with Le Fort 1 osteotomy, BSSO, and genioplasty

Explanation: This patient has features consistent with hemimandibular hyperplasia, including three-dimensional enlargement of the mandible, transverse canting of the occlusal plane, and supraeruption of maxillary molars. Given that condylar growth has stopped, the recommended approach is a combination of orthodontics, Le Fort 1 osteotomy, BSSO and genioplasty to correct the asymmetry, realign the mandible, and address occlusal issues. BSSO alone would not correct the maxillary cant. Condylectomy is unnecessary since growth has already ceased. Genioplasty would only improve chin aesthetics without correcting the underlying skeletal and occlusal issues. Reduction of the mandibular inferior border may be considered as an adjunct but would not address the occlusal cant or midline deviation adequately on its own.

Q6. **Low-flow vascular malformations**

Answer: C. Sclerotherapy with sclerosant agents

Explanation: Low-flow vascular malformations, such as venous malformations, are typically treated with interventional radiological techniques like sclerotherapy. Sclerosants such as absolute alcohol, sodium tetradecyl sulfate (STD), or bleomycin are used to reduce the size and symptoms of the lesion. Surgery is reserved for cases where debulking or excision is necessary, but it has a minor role. Pulsed dye laser therapy is more appropriate for superficial capillary malformations, and embolisation is used for high-flow AVMs, not low-flow venous malformations. Observation is not appropriate for symptomatic or progressively enlarging lesions.

Q7. **Timing of cleft palate repair**

Answer: A. To support speech and language development

Explanation: The timing of cleft palate repair is chosen to balance the requirements of speech development with considerations for maxillary growth. Performing the surgery at approximately 12 months is optimal, as delaying beyond this point can negatively impact speech, increasing the likelihood of velopharyngeal insufficiency and disrupting normal phonation. Early palate closure facilitates proper speech development, while postponing the procedure risks complications with maxillary growth. Although other factors are relevant, they are secondary to the critical need for supporting speech development during this period.

Q8. **Unilateral cleft lip repair**

Answer: B. Realignment of the orbicularis oris

Explanation: A successful unilateral cleft lip repair focuses on restoring the orbicularis oris muscle to its proper anatomical alignment. This ensures the muscle's continuity across the lip, promoting symmetrical movement and avoiding deformities such as a whistling lip. While techniques like nasal base augmentation contribute to aesthetics, proper muscle realignment is essential for restoring functional outcomes. Realigning the orbicularis oris allows for effective speech, facial expression, and oral competence.

Q9. **Vomer flap**

Answer: C. To establish continuity of the nasal floor

Explanation: In bilateral cleft lip and palate repair, the vomer flap plays a crucial role in creating a continuous nasal floor. This is a vital step in preventing oral-nasal fistulas and ensuring proper separation between the oral and nasal cavities. While long-term goals include maintaining maxillary growth and preventing fistulas, the primary early objective of the vomer flap is to secure nasal floor continuity, providing stability and functional support to the midface.

Q10. **Hemifacial microsomia**

Answer: C. Placement of a tracheostomy and feeding tube

Explanation: In severe cases of hemifacial microsomia with mandibular hypoplasia, breathing and feeding can be compromised. The primary management focus is to secure the airway and ensure adequate nutrition. In such cases, placement of a tracheostomy and feeding tube is often necessary to address immediate functional needs. A long line and TPN may be beneficial in the short term but would not address the breathing issues. Mandibular lengthening using distraction osteogenesis may be considered later but is not typically the first intervention for a young child with acute respiratory and feeding issues. Ear reconstruction, orthognathic surgery, and malar augmentation are cosmetic and structural interventions that are usually postponed until the patient is older and growth is closer to completion.

Q11. **High-flow vascular malformations**

Answer: C. Embolisation followed by surgical resection

Explanation: High-flow AVMs in the mandible require a multidisciplinary approach. Embolisation is used as an initial step to reduce blood flow and minimise intraoperative bleeding. Definitive management involves surgical resection to remove the nidus and reconstruct the defect.

In some cases, surgical resection may not be feasible due to the extent or location of the lesion, and embolisation alone is carried out. However, this approach carries a higher risk of recurrence and the development of collateral vessels, which can complicate future management. For this reason, embolisation alone is generally avoided when a combined approach is possible. Radiation therapy and conservative monitoring are not appropriate for active, symptomatic AVMs.

Q12. **Staging cleft lip and palate repair**

Answer: B. To prevent velopharyngeal insufficiency as speech develops

Explanation: Staging cleft lip and palate repair is essential to optimise speech development and the function of the velopharyngeal mechanism. Lip repair is typically performed first to correct aesthetic and structural issues, while palate repairs are done later to close the oronasal communication, which is crucial for speech. Performing palate repair after lip repair reduces the risk of velopharyngeal insufficiency, which can significantly affect speech. This approach also helps manage maxillary growth and reduce complications like fistula formation, but preventing speech problems remains the primary goal.

Q13. **Secondary alveolar bone grafting**

Answer: C. When the permanent canine's root development is between one-half and two-thirds complete

Explanation: The ideal timing for secondary alveolar bone grafting is when the permanent canine's root has developed between two-thirds and three-fourths, based on radiographic evaluation. This stage ensures the best integration of the graft with the developing dentition, especially in supporting the unerupted canine. Grafting can also be performed earlier if the lateral incisor is still unerupted to support dental arch stability. If the canine has already erupted, bone grafting remains beneficial, but the outcomes may be less favourable compared to performing it earlier when the root is still developing.

Q14. **Fronto-orbital remodelling**

Answer: A. Fronto-orbital remodelling with advancement and calvarial reshaping

Explanation: Fronto-orbital remodelling with advancement corrects both intracranial hypertension and craniofacial deformities in coronal craniosynostosis, addressing orbital dystopia and forehead retrusion. Other options are either insufficient or suited for different craniosynostosis types.

Q15. **Metopic craniosynostosis**

Answer: C. Total cranial vault remodelling surgery

Explanation: In an infant with metopic craniosynostosis, particularly with increased intracranial pressure and developmental delay, total cranial vault remodelling surgery is the most appropriate approach. This procedure corrects the cranial deformity and alleviates pressure on the brain, supporting normal development. Endoscopic strip craniectomy with helmet therapy is typically used for less severe cases without developmental concerns. Cranial distraction is more commonly indicated for syndromic craniosynostosis, and delaying surgery could worsen developmental outcomes.

Q16. **Tessier classification system**

Answer: C. Tessier classification

Explanation: The Tessier classification system is a method used to categorise facial clefts by assigning numbers to different locations of the cleft on the face, ranging from 0 to 14, with lower numbers representing midline clefts and higher numbers indicating more lateral clefts. Clefts numbered 0–7 are considered facial clefts, while 8–14 are classified as cranial clefts. This presentation suggests a midline craniofacial cleft, often associated with holoprosencephaly.

Q17. **Craniofacial cleft management**

Answer: D. Comprehensive soft tissue repair combined with midface skeletal repositioning using a frontofacial monobloc advancement

Explanation: A frontofacial monobloc advancement is the preferred approach for complex craniofacial clefts like Tessier 4, as it corrects both midface asymmetry and functional deformities, including orbital dystopia and nasal deformities. Primary soft tissue repair alone with delayed skeletal correction leads to suboptimal outcomes by failing to address the underlying bony asymmetry. Simultaneous soft tissue repair and midface distraction osteogenesis is more suitable for midface hypoplasia but does not adequately manage the severe skeletal component of Tessier 4 clefts. A staged approach with Le Fort I osteotomy in adolescence is insufficient, as it only advances the maxilla and does not correct orbital or midface deformities. Finally, isolated orbital floor reconstruction with skin grafting addresses only localised defects without treating the broader midface and skeletal abnormalities.

Q18. **Hemifacial microsomia**

Answer: B. Le Fort I osteotomy and active orthodontics

Explanation: In a 13-year-old patient with hemifacial microsomia presenting with maxillary canting, Le Fort I osteotomy combined with active orthodontics can help correct the asymmetry by levelling the maxillary plane. This intervention is typically performed during the later stages of mixed dentition, around the early teenage years, to address developing maxillary canting. Costochondral grafts for mandibular reconstruction or soft tissue augmentation are not indicated as the first intervention in this age group, particularly if the focus is on correcting maxillary asymmetry. Bone-anchored hearing aids are recommended if hearing is affected, but this was not indicated in this case. Observation alone may delay necessary corrective procedures, as some interventions, such as levelling the maxilla, are ideally performed before skeletal maturity.

Q19. **Binder syndrome**

Answer: C. Fusion of the first and second cervical vertebrae

Explanation: The patient's presentation is consistent with Binder syndrome (maxillo-nasal dysplasia), characterised by midfacial hypoplasia, flat nasal bridge, short nose, absent anterior nasal spine, and Class III skeletal and dental profile. Cervical spine anomalies, including fusion of the first and second cervical vertebrae, are commonly associated with Binder syndrome.

- A. Multiple basal cell carcinomas and keratocystic odontogenic tumours are pathognomonic for Gorlin-Goltz syndrome (nevoid basal cell carcinoma syndrome).
- B. Hypocalcaemia and a history of congenital heart defects are features of DiGeorge syndrome (22q11.2 deletion syndrome).
- D. Craniosynostosis with shallow orbits and hypertelorism is characteristic of Crouzon syndrome.
- E. Oral fibrous papules and intestinal hamartomatous polyps are associated with Cowden syndrome.

Q20. **Craniofacial cleft management**

Answer: C. Monobloc advancement with midface and orbital repositioning

Explanation: Monobloc advancement with midface and orbital repositioning is the most appropriate approach for correcting complex orbital dystopia, hypertelorism, and midface hypoplasia in patients with a history of Tessier 3 craniofacial cleft repair. This technique repositions the midface and orbits as a single unit, addressing both functional and aesthetic concerns. Isolated orbital roof reconstruction with titanium mesh is useful for superior orbital defects but does not correct midface involvement. Distraction osteogenesis of the zygomatic complex can improve midface projection but does not effectively reposition the orbit. Osteotomy and orbital floor repositioning with soft tissue adjustment may be suitable for minor vertical orbital displacement but is inadequate for cases with extensive dystopia. Endoscopic medial wall repositioning with alloplastic graft placement is primarily used for medial orbital defects or enophthalmos and does not address the broader facial asymmetry seen in this patient.

Q21. **Embryology of facial clefts**

Answer: A. Fusion of the medial nasal and maxillary prominences

Explanation: Midline facial clefts occur due to a failure of the medial nasal prominences to fuse with the maxillary prominences during embryological development, disrupting normal midface formation. In contrast, failure of the lateral nasal and maxillary prominences to fuse typically results in nasolacrimal duct abnormalities rather than midline defects. Improper formation of the frontal bone from the neural crest affects cranial development but does not directly cause a facial cleft. Fusion failure of the mandibular prominences primarily affects the lower jaw, while incomplete closure of the anterior neuropore leads to severe neural tube defects such as encephalocele or anencephaly rather than isolated midline facial clefts.

Q22. **Treacher-Collins syndrome**

Answer: A. Mutations in the TCOF1 gene

Explanation: Mandibular hypoplasia, auricular deformity, and an epibulbar dermoid in a child with a de novo mutation are characteristic of Treacher-Collins syndrome, which is most commonly associated with mutations in the *TCOF1* gene. This condition, a form of craniofacial microsomia, affects the development of the first and second pharyngeal arches. In contrast, a chromosome 22q11.2 deletion is linked to DiGeorge syndrome, which primarily presents with cardiac and thymic defects. *FGFR2* mutations are associated with craniosynostosis syndromes like Apert and Crouzon syndromes, which involve premature fusion of cranial sutures rather than mandibular hypoplasia. Pathogenic variants in *EYA1* cause Branchio-Oto-Renal syndrome, which involves branchial arch anomalies and renal abnormalities but not craniofacial microsomia. Mutations in *SALL4* are seen in Duane Radial Ray syndrome, a disorder affecting limb and ocular development without significant mandibular involvement.

Q23. **Primary neurulation**

Answer: B. Primary neurulation

Explanation: A midline scalp defect containing neural tissue in a 3-month-old is most likely due to failed primary neurulation, a crucial process in early embryogenesis that occurs within the first four weeks and can lead to neural tube defects such as encephaloceles. This differs from defects in neural crest migration, which primarily affect cranial bone development without causing neural herniation. Failure of secondary palate fusion results in cleft palate rather than skull defects. Improper somite differentiation into sclerotomes impacts vertebral development rather than the calvarium. Additionally, failure of posterior neuropore closure leads to spinal defects like myelomeningocele rather than cranial abnormalities.

Q24. **Neurofibromatosis Type 1**

Answer: A. Mutation in the NF1 gene on chromosome 17

Explanation: Neurofibromatosis Type 1 (NF1) is caused by a mutation in the NF1 gene on chromosome 17 and is characterised by café-au-lait macules, axillary freckling, and plexiform neurofibromas, as seen in this patient. In contrast, NF2 gene mutations on chromosome 22 lead to Neurofibromatosis Type 2, which is associated with bilateral vestibular schwannomas rather than plexiform neurofibromas. PTEN gene deletions on chromosome 10 cause Cowden syndrome, presenting with multiple hamartomas and an increased malignancy risk. TP53 mutations result in Li-Fraumeni syndrome, which predisposes individuals to various early-onset cancers. Chromosome 22q11 deletion is linked to DiGeorgevelocardiofacial syndrome, which primarily affects the craniofacial and cardiovascular systems.

Q25. **Chiari malformation**

Answer: B. Obstruction of CSF flow

Explanation: Chiari malformation occurs when cerebellar tonsillar herniation impedes CSF flow, leading to increased intracranial pressure and symptoms like headaches and ataxia. Excessive production of CSF is rare and typically associated with conditions like choroid plexus papilloma.

Q26. **Secondary cleft rhinoplasty**

Answer: B. Correcting nasal asymmetry and septal deviation

Explanation: Secondary cleft rhinoplasty addresses both functional (airway) and aesthetic (nasal symmetry, tip projection).concerns

Q27. **Classification systems post alveolar bone graft to cleft lip and palate**

Answer: B. Bergland Grade II

Explanation:

- **Bergland Grade II** is the correct classification, as the bone level is >75% of the normal contralateral side.
- **Chelsea Category F (C)**: Refers to a bony bridge with 25% or less coverage, which does not align with the described radiographic findings.
- **Kindelan Grade 3 (D)**: Represents <50% bony infill, which is inconsistent with the reported 80%.
- **Kindelan Grade 4 (E)**: Indicates no bony bridge and is classified as a failure, which is also incorrect in this context.

Q28. **Velopharyngeal insufficiency management**

Answer: C. Bilateral posterior pharyngeal flaps to narrow the velopharyngeal gap

Explanation: Orticochea pharyngoplasty involves bilateral posterior pharyngeal flaps to create a dynamic sphincter. This technique is ideal for patients with lateral wall motion deficits.

Q29. **Velopharyngeal insufficiency management**

Answer: C. Furlow double-opposing Z-plasty

Explanation: Furlow palatoplasty is ideal for treating VPI with a small gap by lengthening the soft palate and improving velopharyngeal closure. It is particularly effective for speech improvement.

Q30. **Secondary alveolar bone graft**

Answer: B. Secondary alveolar bone graft

Explanation: Secondary alveolar bone grafting is typically performed before the eruption of the permanent canine when its root development is between two-thirds and three-quarters. This procedure provides structural support for the canine and addresses the palatal fistula.

Q31. **Staging of cleft palate treatment**

Answer: C. Palatoplasty to repair the cleft and improve speech

Explanation: At 12 months, palatoplasty is typically performed to close the cleft and restore velopharyngeal function for speech. Delaying repair increases the risk of speech and feeding difficulties. Alveolar bone grafting is performed later, usually before the eruption of the permanent canine.

Q32. **22q11.2 Deletion syndrome**

Answer: B. Thymic hypoplasia leading to immunodeficiency

Explanation: 22q11.2 Deletion syndrome (DiGeorge/velocardiofacial syndrome) is a genetic disorder characterised by thymic hypoplasia, leading to T-cell immunodeficiency, along with parathyroid hypoplasia (causing hypocalcaemia), cardiac anomalies, and craniofacial features such as cleft palate and velopharyngeal insufficiency. Bilateral microtia and conductive hearing loss would be seen in other conditions such as Treacher-Collins syndrome. Retinal detachment due to connective tissue disorder is a feature of Stickler syndrome, not 22q11.2 deletion syndrome.

Q33. **Airway management**

Answer: B. Place a nasopharyngeal airway

Explanation: Initial management of airway obstruction in Pierre Robin sequence involves positioning and use of a nasopharyngeal airway to alleviate glossoptosis-induced airway obstruction. Gastrostomy and tracheostomy may be required but would not be the next step.

Q34. **Stickler syndrome**

Answer: B. Mutation in the COL2A1 gene

Explanation: Stickler Syndrome is a connective tissue disorder caused by mutations in the COL2A1 gene, leading to features such as midface hypoplasia, cleft palate, hearing loss, and ocular abnormalities (e.g., myopia, retinal detachment).

Q35. **Velopharyngeal insufficiency**

Answer: D. Velopharyngeal insufficiency

Explanation: Hypernasal speech and nasal air emission are hallmark signs of velopharyngeal insufficiency (VPI), where the repaired palate fails to achieve adequate closure against the posterior pharyngeal wall during speech.

Q36. **Oronasal fistula**

Answer: C. Oronasal fistula

Explanation: Oronasal fistulae are a common complication of cleft palate repair, especially along the repair suture lines. These fistulae result in nasal regurgitation and can interfere with swallowing.

Q37. **Tensor veli palatini**

Answer: A. Dysfunction of the tensor veli palatini muscle

Explanation: The tensor veli palatini muscle plays a critical role in opening the eustachian tube during swallowing. Dysfunction due to cleft palate repair often leads to middle ear effusion and recurrent otitis media, resulting in conductive hearing loss. During cleft palate repair, it's recommended to avoid releasing the TVP tendon from the hamulus. Scarring of the eustachian tube would also explain the symptoms but should not be a direct complication of the surgery.

Q38. **Functional abnormalities due to cleft lip and palate**

Answer: D. Inability to generate suction due to palatal defect

Explanation: The cleft palate prevents effective suction by disrupting the separation of the oral and nasal cavities, leading to a failure to create negative pressure during feeding.

Q39. **Velopharyngeal insufficiency management**

Answer: B. Sphincter pharyngoplasty

Explanation: Sphincter pharyngoplasty is the operation of choice for patients with a coronal or circular closure pattern, especially when lateral wall motion is strong, but palatal motion is limited. Pharyngeal flap surgery is best for patients with good lateral wall motion but a large midline gap. Furlow palatoplasty is suitable for sagittal closure patterns or patients with a small midline palatal gap. Posterior pharyngeal wall augmentation can be used in select cases of small velopharyngeal gaps. Speech therapy may be helpful as adjunctive therapy but is not sufficient to address significant anatomical VPI.

Q40. **Van der Woude syndrome**

Answer: B. Van der Woude syndrome

Explanation: Van der Woude syndrome is the most common syndromic cause of cleft lip and/or palate, characterised by clefts and lower lip pits. It follows an autosomal dominant inheritance pattern due to mutations in the IRF6 gene. Pits are found at the junction of the wet and dry of the vermillion and are blind ended traversing through orbicularis oris. Hypodontia is a common feature. Extraoral features are rare and include heart defects, accessory nipple, popliteal web, and Hirschsprung disease. Pierre Robin sequence also commonly features cleft lip and palate. The frequency of occurrence of various deformities are micrognathia (91.7%), glossoptosis (70%–85%) or macroglossia and ankyloglossia (10%–15%) and cleft palate (14%) (16, 17).

Q41. **Staging of treatment for cleft lip and palate**

Answer: D. Definitive lip repair

Explanation: Definitive lip repair is typically performed between 3 and 6 months of age, following the "Rule of 10s" (initially reported by Wilhelmsen and Musgrave (1966) and Millard (1976), surgery should be delayed until the patient is 10 weeks old, weighs >10 pounds, Hb >10 g/l, and a white cell count of <10,000 cells/cc). Palate repair is delayed until 9–18 months to reduce the impact on midfacial growth and allow for speech development.

Q42. **Embryology of cleft lip**

Answer: C. Failure of maxillary and medial nasal processes to merge

Explanation: A unilateral cleft lip occurs due to the failure of the maxillary and medial nasal processes to merge during the fourth to seventh week of embryonic development. This is distinct from cleft palate, which involves disruption in the formation or fusion of the palatal shelves. Lateral nasal processes contribute to the alar of the nose.

Q43. **Positional plagiocephaly**

Answer: D. Tummy time and positional changes are the first-line management.

Explanation: This child presents with positional plagiocephaly, characterised by posterior skull flattening, forward displacement of the ipsilateral ear, and ipsilateral frontal bossing. It results from external pressure on the skull, typically due to a preferred head position. Management is conservative with tummy time and positional changes, as the condition tends to improve naturally. Helmet therapy is controversial, with limited evidence of benefit, and surgical correction is not indicated because this is a non-synostotic condition. Unlike lambdoid synostosis, positional plagiocephaly is not associated with premature suture fusion, and it does not predispose to facial or TMJ abnormalities. Differentiating the two conditions is essential for appropriate management.

Q44. **Functional abnormalities due to cleft lip and palate**

Answer: D. Distortions or substitutions of plosives such as "p" and "b" may occur.

Explanation: Unilateral cleft lip causes structural and functional abnormalities that can lead to speech difficulties. Distortions or substitutions of plosives such as "p" and "b" are common due to the inability to generate sufficient intraoral pressure. Anatomically, Cupid's bow is rotated towards the cleft side (left), and the philtral column is shortened on the cleft side. The nasal tip is deflected to the contralateral side (right) and flattened due to underlying nasal cartilage deformation. Additionally, the nasal septum is often deviated in unilateral cleft lip cases, contributing to nasal asymmetry.

Q45. **Tennison-Randall approach**

Answer: B. A triangular flap based laterally is used to fill the deficiency in lip height, with a back-cut extending from the cleft Cupid's bow peak toward the centre of the philtrum.

Explanation: The Tennison-Randall technique is a geometric-based repair that involves a back-cut from the cleft Cupid's bow peak toward the centre of the philtrum, followed by a laterally based triangular flap that has width equal to the measured deficiency in lip height. Two points of closure along the nostril floor are designed so that when they are brought together, the nasal deformity is corrected. From these two points, corresponding lines are dropped to the cleft Cupid's bow peak medially and to the base of the triangular flap laterally. This design helps address both the vertical deficiency of the lip and the nasal deformity associated with wide clefts. The technique utilises precise anatomic landmarks and calipers to guide the design, which is essential in ensuring both functional and aesthetic outcomes, particularly in cases of severe vertical deficiency. While the approach aims for symmetry, it has been criticised for occasionally resulting in lips that are too long if the lateral lip element is not shortened appropriately (18).

Q46. **Millard approach**

Answer: B. A curvilinear incision extends from the Cupid's bow peak toward the noncleft philtral column, allowing for rotation and advancement to correct the cleft deformity.

Explanation: The Millard approach is a rotation-advancement repair designed to preserve the philtral dimple and respect anatomic borders. A curvilinear incision is made from the Cupid's bow peak on the cleft side toward the noncleft philtral column. The rotation of the medial lip, along with advancement of the lateral lip, corrects the cleft deformity. The lateral lip advancement also helps in narrowing the nostril floor and correcting the alar flare. A superiorly based C-flap is then used for nasal floor closure. For the Mohler modification, a rotation incision is designed to mirror the normal philtral column and extends onto the columella. A back-cut is designed to end at the lip-columellar junction, and the C-flap is used to both fill the columellar defect and abut the rotated lip segment. Lip closure follows anatomic subunits (19).

8 TMJ and Orthognathic

QUESTIONS

Q1. Which of the following is true regarding TMJ arthroscopy?
   A. The first puncture point is located 10 mm anterior to the tragus and 5 mm above the cananthotragal line.
   B. Level I arthroscopy involves multiple punctures for advanced operative procedures, such as discopropexy.
   C. The seven points of visualisation include the articular disc and retrodiscal synovium.
   D. The second puncture point for the outflow needle is 15 mm anterior and 5 mm above the trabugus.
   E. Level III arthroscopy is diagnostic and limited to arthrocentesis.

Q2. Which of the following statements about TMJ arthroscopy is true?
   A. Platelet-rich plasma (PRP) used in TMJ arthroscopy must always be activated by thrombin and calcium chloride to achieve its therapeutic effects.
   B. Hyaluronic acid (HA) improves TMJ function by directly stimulating synovial fluid production.
   C. Otological complications during TMJ arthroscopy are most commonly caused by perforation of the tympanic membrane.
   D. Extravasation of irrigation fluid into the parapharyngeal space may delay extubation and require monitoring.
   E. Arthroscopic discopexy has higher complication rates compared to an open approach due to the proximity of the middle cranial fossa.

Q3. A 29-year-old woman undergoes injections to address a square-shaped jawline and muscle discomfort in her cheeks, especially during chewing. Which of the following describes the primary mechanism of action of this treatment?
   A. Irreversibly binds to acetylcholine channels
   B. Blocks voltage-gated sodium channels
   C. Acts as an agonist at GABA receptors, increasing inhibitory neurotransmission
   D. Cleaves SNAP-25
   E. Inhibits norepinephrine reuptake at adrenergic nerve terminals

Q4. A 25-year-old male presents with limited mandibular opening due to ankylosis of the temporomandibular joint. Imaging reveals mild condylar irregularities but no significant bone destruction. What is the primary indication for a condylar shave in this case?
   A. Correct occlusal discrepancies
   B. Relieve joint ankylosis and restore motion
   C. Prevent recurrence of ankylosis

DOI: 10.1201/9781003609308-9

D. Reduce pain associated with TMJ arthritis
E. Address facial asymmetry

Q5. A 29-year-old female with TMJ clicking and mild pain is diagnosed with anterior disc displacement with reduction. She underwent level 2 arthroscopy six months ago without benefit. Which of the following if most appropriate?
A. Eminectomy
B. Condylar shave
C. Disc plication
D. Discectomy
E. Arthrocentesis

Q6. A 25-year-old patient presents with crowding in the lower anterior teeth. Cephalometric analysis shows a mandibular incisor inclination (LInc to MnPl) of 100°. How would this measurement be interpreted in terms of mandibular incisor positioning?
A. Within the normal range, indicating no significant incisor inclination
B. Increased inclination, indicating labial tipping of mandibular incisors
C. Decreased inclination, indicating lingual tipping of mandibular incisors
D. Increased inclination, indicating lingual tipping of mandibular incisors
E. Decreased inclination, indicating labial tipping of mandibular incisors

Q7. A 28-year-old patient presents with a bird-face deformity characterised by significant retrogenia, a concave facial profile, and mandibular retrognathism. The patient has a Class I occlusion and no functional dental issues. What is the most appropriate management?
A. Maxillary advancement surgery
B. Maxillary setback surgery and mandibular advancement with genioplasty
C. Orthodontic treatment alone
D. Mandibular advancement with genioplasty
E. Distraction osteogenesis of the mandible

Q8. A 14-year-old patient presents with a prominent maxillary dental arch, increased overjet, retrognathic mandible, and a normal maxillomandibular plane angle (MMPA). The patient is being evaluated for orthognathic surgery. What is the most appropriate management option?
A. Maxillary impaction surgery with mandibular autorotation
B. Orthodontic alignment followed by mandibular advancement surgery
C. Orthodontic conversion to Class II Division 2 malocclusion and mandibular setback
D. Mandibular distraction osteogenesis
E. Orthodontic alignment alone

Q9. A 17-year-old patient presents with a Class II Division 2 malocclusion, characterised by retroclined maxillary incisors, a deep overbite, and a short lower facial height. The patient has a skeletal Class II pattern with mandibular retrusion. Orthodontic alignment has been completed, and the patient is being evaluated for orthognathic surgery. What is the most appropriate surgical intervention?

A. Bilateral sagittal split osteotomy with mandibular advancement and orthodontic camouflage
B. Bilateral sagittal split osteotomy with mandibular advancement to a three-point landing
C. Surgically assisted rapid palatal expansion
D. Segmental maxillary osteotomy
E. Bimaxillary surgery with maxillary advancement and mandibular setback

Q10. Which of the following is the most appropriate indication for total TMJ replacement?
A. Anterior disc displacement without reduction
B. Osteoarthritis unresponsive to conservative therapy
C. Bilateral condylar hyperplasia
D. Ankylosis with significant functional impairment
E. Recurrent dislocation

Q11. A 25-year-old male presents with restricted jaw opening and joint discomfort three months after undergoing a bilateral sagittal split osteotomy for mandibular advancement. Imaging reveals malpositioned condyles with anterior displacement in the glenoid fossa. What is the most likely cause of this complication?
A. Over-tightening of fixation plates
B. Inadequate proximal segment seating during surgery
C. Condylar resorption
D. Incomplete osteotomy of the mandibular ramus
E. Excessive mandibular advancement beyond 10 mm

Q12. A 22-year-old male undergoing orthognathic surgery is assessed using cephalometric analysis. His SNA angle measures 78° and SNB angle measures 82°. Which of the following would be a suitable treatment plan?
A. Mandibular setback
B. Bimaxillary surgery
C. Maxillary advancement only
D. Orthodontics camouflage
E. Observation and regular follow-up

Q13. A 24-year-old male with vertical maxillary excess presents with excessive gingival show on smiling and long face syndrome. He undergoes preoperative assessment for orthognathic surgery, including cephalometric analysis, which confirms vertical maxillary hyperplasia with normal mandibular positioning. Which of the following procedures would be the most stable postoperatively?
A. Maxillary advancement
B. Mandibular advancement
C. Maxillary posterior impaction
D. Mandibular setback
E. Bimaxillary surgery

Q14. A 21-year-old female undergoes bimaxillary surgery for correction of a Class III malocclusion. At her six-month postoperative review, a mild anterior open bite has developed despite radiographic evidence of stable fixation. Which of the following factors is most likely responsible for this relapse?

A. Excessive clockwise rotation of the maxilla during surgery
B. Inadequate orthodontic decompensation preoperatively
C. Condylar resorption leading to posterior mandibular rotation
D. Muscular and soft tissue tension opposing skeletal changes
E. Poor postoperative elastic management

Q15. A 14-year-old male presents with a Class II Division 1 malocclusion. Which of the following best describes this classification?
A. Lower first molar is mesially positioned relative to the upper first molar, with retroclined upper incisors
B. Lower first molar is distally positioned relative to the upper first molar, with retroclined upper incisors
C. Lower first molar is distally positioned relative to the upper first molar, with proclined upper incisors
D. Lower first molar is mesially positioned relative to the upper first molar, with proclined upper incisors
E. Lower first molar is in normal relationship with the upper first molar, with proclined upper incisors

Q16. A 15-year-old girl presents with an anterior open bite and significant vertical maxillary excess. Which of the following is the most likely contributing factor?
A. Unilateral condylar hyperplasia
B. Mouth breathing due to chronic nasal obstruction
C. Unilateral temporomandibular joint ankylosis
D. Hemi-facial microsomia
E. Submucous cleft palate

Q17. A 17-year-old female presents with progressive mandibular asymmetry. Examination reveals chin deviation to the left and a crossbite on the right side. Imaging confirms increased vertical height of the right mandibular condyle. What is the most appropriate next step in management?
A. Perform mandibular condylectomy immediately
B. Initiate orthodontic treatment to correct the crossbite
C. Tc-99 m-MDP bone scintigraphy to evaluate condylar growth activity
D. FDG PET to assess condylar growth activity
E. Repeat imaging in six months

Q18. A 25-year-old man visits the orthognathic clinic for evaluation of a receding chin. Cephalometric analysis reveals a retrognathic chin with the pogonion positioned 10 mm behind the ideal facial line. He has a normal occlusion with no significant dental misalignment. What is the most suitable surgical option to address his aesthetic concern?
A. Sliding genioplasty with posterior repositioning
B. Alloplastic chin augmentation
C. Maxillary advancement using Le Fort I osteotomy
D. Bilateral sagittal split osteotomy
E. Mandibular setback

Q19. A 17-year-old male with a history of obstructive sleep apnoea (OSA) seeks an orthognathic assessment. He previously underwent adenotonsillectomy, which provided limited improvement. Cephalometric analysis shows a maxillary deficiency and a Class III skeletal pattern. His apnoea-hypopnea index (AHI) is still high at 40 events per hour. What is the most appropriate surgical treatment option?
A. Maxillary advancement with mandibular setback
B. Maxillary advancement using Le Fort I osteotomy
C. Genioplasty with anterior repositioning
D. Bilateral sagittal split osteotomy (BSSO) for mandibular advancement
E. Maxillary expansion using distraction osteogenesis

ANSWERS AND EXPLANATIONS

Q1. **TMJ arthroscopy**

Answer: C. The seven points of visualisation include the articular disc and retrodiscal synovium.

Explanation: TMJ arthroscopy provides detailed visualisation of intra-articular structures (20), including the seven points of visualisation: (1) medial synovial drape, (2) pterygoid shadow, (3) retrodiscal synovium, (4) posterior slope of the articular eminence and glenoid fossa, (5) articular disc, (6) intermediate zone, and (7) anterior recess.

The first puncture point is correctly located 10 mm anterior to the tragus and 2 mm below the canthotragal line. The second puncture point for the outflow needle is 20 mm anterior to the tragus and 10 mm below the line (Holmlund-Hellsing line).

Arthroscopy levels are classified as follows:

- Level I arthroscopy is single-puncture diagnostic arthroscopy with arthrocentesis.
- Level II arthroscopy involves double-puncture operative arthroscopy, allowing for procedures such as biopsy and debridement.
- Level III arthroscopy is the most advanced, involving multiple punctures for procedures like discopexy or managing mandibular dislocation.

Q2. **TMJ arthroscopy**

Answer: D. Extravasation of irrigation fluid into the parapharyngeal space may delay extubation and require monitoring.

Explanation: Extravasation of irrigation fluid is the most common complication of TMJ arthroscopy. While it is typically benign and resolves spontaneously, fluid accumulation in the parapharyngeal space can occasionally delay extubation and necessitate prolonged monitoring.

- A. PRP is not always activated by thrombin and calcium chloride; these are used for plasma rich in growth factors (PRGF) to create a fibrin gel for targeted delivery, but PRP itself can still be effective without activation.
- B. Hyaluronic acid (HA) does not directly stimulate synovial fluid production; its benefits are associated with increasing viscosity and elasticity of the synovial fluid, reducing pain, and improving joint mobility.
- C. Otological complications are most commonly due to extravasation of irrigation fluid into the middle ear, not tympanic membrane perforation. Patients may experience symptoms such as hearing loss, tinnitus, or vertigo.

- E. Arthroscopic discopexy has lower complication rates compared to open approaches. Its advantages include smaller incisions, reduced operating time, guided injections, and reduced risk of complications like bleeding or infections.

Q3. **Botulinum toxin**

Answer: D. Cleaves SNAP-25

Explanation: Botulinum toxin (BoNT) injections work by specifically targeting the SNARE complex in cholinergic nerve terminals, which is essential for the release of acetylcholine, the main neurotransmitter at the neuromuscular junction. BoNT binds to the presynaptic surface of cholinergic nerve terminals and enters the neuron through endocytosis. BoNT interacts with the SNARE complex, which includes synaptobrevin, SNAP-25, and syntaxin. Different BoNT serotypes cleave different components of the SNARE complex. BoNT-A cleaves SNAP-25. The cleavage of the SNARE complex prevents the release of acetylcholine, which is the main neurotransmitter at the neuromuscular junction. The muscle is chemically denervated, meaning it can't contract., which is why it is effective in treating masseteric hypertrophy.

The other options describe mechanisms of action for different classes of drugs:

- Blocks voltage-gated sodium channels on muscle fibres: This is the mechanism of action for local anaesthetics, which block nerve signal conduction.
- Acts as an agonist at GABA receptors, increasing inhibitory neurotransmission: This describes the mechanism of action of certain sedatives, like benzodiazepines, which enhance GABA-mediated inhibition.
- Inhibits norepinephrine reuptake at adrenergic nerve terminals: This mechanism is associated with certain antidepressants and stimulant medications, which increase norepinephrine availability.

Q4. **Condylar shave**

Answer: B. Relieve joint ankylosis and restore motion

Explanation: Condylar shaving is used to remove fibrous adhesions or bony irregularities causing restricted motion, especially in early ankylosis.

Q5. **Disc plication**

Answer: C. Disc plication

Explanation: Disc plication repositions the displaced disc and secures it in the correct position, improving joint function and reducing symptoms in cases of reducible disc displacement.

Q6. **Cephalometric analysis**

Answer: B. Increased inclination, indicating labial tipping of mandibular incisors

Explanation: The normal range for mandibular incisor inclination (LInc to MnPl) is 93° ± 6°. A value of 100° exceeds this range, indicating an increased inclination. This suggests labial tipping of the mandibular incisors, which may be associated with crowding and proclination in the lower anterior region.

Refresher guide for cephalometric analysis:
Cephalometric Points

1. ***A Point (A)*** *– Deepest concavity on the maxillary alveolus (anteriorly).*
2. ***B Point (B)*** *– Deepest concavity on the mandibular symphysis (anteriorly).*

3. ***Sella (S)*** *– Midpoint of the sella turcica (pituitary fossa).*
4. ***Nasion (N)*** *– Most anterior point on the fronto-nasal suture.*
5. ***Orbitale (Or)*** *– Most anterior, inferior point on the infraorbital rim.*
6. ***Porion (Po)*** *– Upper midpoint on the external auditory meatus.*
7. ***Anterior Nasal Spine (ANS)*** *– Tip of the anterior nasal spine.*
8. ***Posterior Nasal Spine (PNS)*** *– Tip of the posterior nasal spine.*
9. ***Gonion (Go)*** *– Most posterior, inferior point on the mandibular angle.*
10. ***Gnathion (Gn)*** *– Most anterior, inferior point on the mandibular symphysis.*
11. ***Menton (Me)*** *– Most inferior point on the mandibular symphysis.*
12. ***Pogonion (Pog)*** *– Most anterior point on the mandibular symphysis.*

Cephalometric Planes and Relationships

1. ***SN Line*** *– A plane through the nasion and sella, used as a cranial base reference.*
2. ***Frankfort Plane*** *– A plane through the orbitale and porion, representing a horizontal reference.*
3. ***Mandibular Plane (MnPl)*** *– A line through the gonion and menton, showing the plane of the mandible's lower border.*
4. ***Maxillary Plane (MxPl)*** *– A line through the anterior and posterior nasal spines, representing the plane of the maxilla.*

Key Angles

1. ***SNA*** *– Angle representing the anteroposterior position of the maxilla relative to the cranial base.*
2. ***SNB*** *– Angle representing the anteroposterior position of the mandible relative to the cranial base.*
3. ***ANB*** *– Angle representing the anteroposterior relationship between the maxilla and mandible, used for skeletal classification.*
4. ***Inter-incisal Angle*** *– The angle between the long axis of the maxillary and mandibular incisors.*
5. ***Maxillary-Mandibular Plane Angle (MMPA)*** *– Angle between the maxillary and mandibular planes.*
6. ***Maxillary Incisal Inclination (UInc to MxPl)*** *– Angle between the maxillary plane and the axis of the maxillary incisors.*
7. ***Mandibular Incisal Inclination (LInc to MnPl)*** *– Angle between the mandibular plane and the axis of the mandibular incisors.*

Average Values in Cephalometric Analysis Eastman Cephalometric Standards

Angle/Measurement	Average Value
SNA	81° ± 3°
SNB	78° ± 3°
ANB	3° ± 2°
UInc to MxPl	109° ± 6°
LInc to MnPl	93° ± 6°
Inter-Incisal Angle	135° ± 10°
MMPA	27° ± 4°
Facial Proportion	55% ± 2%

Q7. **Common orthognathic patterns**

Answer: D. Mandibular advancement with genioplasty

Explanation: In patients with a bird-face deformity and significant mandibular retrognathism but a Class I occlusion, the appropriate treatment focuses on correcting the facial profile without altering the occlusion. Mandibular advancement with genioplasty addresses both the retrognathism and retrogenia, enhancing the aesthetics of the lower face. Inverted 'L' osteotomies or distraction osteogenesis may be considered in severe cases.

Q8. **Common orthognathic patterns**

Answer: B. Orthodontic alignment followed by mandibular advancement surgery

Explanation: For a Class II Division 1 patient with retrognathic mandible and normal MMPA, the most appropriate treatment involves orthodontic alignment to optimise dental positioning followed by mandibular advancement surgery. This corrects the skeletal discrepancy, establishes a Class I occlusion, and maintains the facial proportions. Maxillary impaction is indicated for Class II patients with a long face and anterior open bite.

Q9. **Common orthognathic patterns**

Answer: B. Bilateral sagittal split osteotomy with mandibular advancement to a three-point landing

Explanation: For Class II Division 2 patients with mandibular retrusion, deep overbite, and reduced lower anterior face height, mandibular advancement to a three-point landing using BSSO is the most appropriate surgical approach. This technique corrects the skeletal discrepancy, increases lower anterior face height, and restores a balanced profile.

Q10. **TMJ replacement**

Answer: D. Ankylosis with significant functional impairment

Explanation: Total TMJ replacement is indicated for ankylosis with severe functional limitations or intractable pain unresponsive to other treatments.

Q11. **Complications of orthognathic surgery**

Answer: B. Inadequate proximal segment seating during surgery

Explanation: Malpositioning of the condyles is often caused by improper seating of the proximal segment during orthognathic surgery. This can result in anterior or posterior displacement, leading to temporomandibular joint dysfunction or condylar resorption in the future

Q12. **Common orthognathic patterns**

Answer: B. Bimaxillary surgery

Explanation: The cephalometric values indicate a Class III skeletal relationship (ANB = −4°, with SNB > SNA). Mandibular setback would be effective for isolated mandibular prognathism, it may not suffice when maxillary hypoplasia coexists, as suggested by the low SNA angle. As a result, bimaxillary surgery would be a better response. Similarly, Maxillary advancement may only improve occlusion partially but would not fully address mandibular prominence.

Q13. **Proffit's hierarchy of stability**

Answer: C. Maxillary posterior impaction

Explanation: According to Proffit's hierarchy of stability, maxillary posterior impaction is the most stable orthognathic procedure, as it benefits from strong bony support and minimal relapse due to soft tissue or muscular forces. This is particularly effective for correcting vertical maxillary excess and anterior open bite.

- **A. Maxillary advancement**: Moderately stable for correcting horizontal maxillary deficiencies but not suitable for this deformity.
- **B. Mandibular advancement**: More suited for Class II skeletal deformities with less stability than posterior impaction.
- **D. Mandibular setback**: The least stable due to relapse forces and inappropriate for vertical issues.
- **E. Bimaxillary surgery**: Stability depends on the movements performed, but posterior impaction alone offers the highest stability for this patient's specific deformity.

Q14. **Complications of orthognathic surgery**

Answer: D. Muscular and soft tissue tension opposing skeletal changes

Explanation: Muscular and soft tissue tension, particularly from the tongue and masticatory muscles, is a primary cause of relapse after skeletal surgeries like bimaxillary procedures. These forces resist the repositioned skeletal framework, especially in cases of anterior open bite or mandibular setbacks.

- **A**: Excessive clockwise rotation of the maxilla would present earlier and be evident postoperatively.
- **B**: Inadequate orthodontic decompensation impacts occlusion more than skeletal stability.
- **C**: Condylar resorption is rare and usually involves joint symptoms with severe relapse.
- **E**: Poor elastic management affects occlusion rather than skeletal positioning.

Q15. **Angle's classification of malocclusion**

Answer: C. Lower first molar is distally positioned relative to the upper first molar, with proclined upper incisors

Explanation: Class II Division 1 malocclusion is defined by a distal positioning of the lower first molar relative to the upper first molar and proclined upper incisors, resulting in increased overjet.

Q16. **Aetiology of anterior open bite**

Answer: B. Mouth breathing due to chronic nasal obstruction

Explanation: Chronic mouth breathing due to nasal obstruction can result in vertical maxillary overgrowth and an anterior open bite due to altered tongue posture and orofacial muscle imbalance (21).

Q17. **Condylar hyperplasia**

Answer: E. Repeat imaging in six months

Explanation: Condylar hyperplasia is characterised by excessive and asymmetric growth of the mandibular condyle. Post-puberty, there is ongoing growth and mandibular changes, but this is largely complete by the beginning of the 3rd decade (22).

Although scintigraphy has been documented as useful in assessing active growth, the current literature base still reports significant drawbacks; as of yet, it has not superseded serial imaging. This is particularly relevant to this question as the patient is 17. In an older patient, it may be of greater use (23).

Q18. **Common orthognathic patterns**

Answer: B. Alloplastic chin augmentation

Explanation: For a patient with a retrognathic chin and normal occlusion, the most appropriate treatment for aesthetic enhancement is usually alloplastic chin augmentation or sliding genioplasty with anterior repositioning. Le Fort I osteotomy or sagittal split osteotomy would not correct the chin deficiency in the absence of malocclusion, and posterior repositioning is not appropriate. Alloplastic chin augmentation offers a less invasive option for improving the chin profile.

Q19. **Obstructive sleep apnoea (OSA)**

Answer: B. Maxillary advancement using Le Fort I osteotomy

Explanation: For patients with OSA and maxillary deficiency, the most appropriate surgical intervention is maxillary advancement using a Le Fort I osteotomy. This procedure increases the airway space by moving the maxilla forward, improving the severity of OSA, and addressing the skeletal discrepancy. Maxillary advancement with mandibular setback (Option A) could worsen the airway obstruction, making it less suitable. Mandibular advancement may also be required (i.e. maxillomandibular advancement) but of the options available B is the single best answer.

9 Facial Aesthetics

QUESTIONS

Q1. A 64-year-old male with a history of hypertension, hypercholesterolemia, hidradenitis suppurativa, rosacea, and asthma presents with concerns about the bumpy enlargement of his nose. He reports significant psychological distress due to his distorted nasal appearance, and states he is unable to go out in public. On examination, he has prominent follicular openings, thickened skin, and a grossly enlarged, nodular nasal contour. Which of the following would be the most effective treatment for this patient?
   A. Topical metronidazole gel
   B. Oral isotretinoin
   C. Dermabrasion
   D. Chemical peel
   E. Surgical debulking

Q2. A 35-year-old female is undergoing laser treatment for facial telangiectasia. The laser wavelength used is 532 nm, and the targeted chromophore is oxyhaemoglobin. Which of the following lasers is this describing?
   A. CO_2 laser
   B. Pulsed dye laser
   C. Potassium Titanyl Phosphate (KTP) laser
   D. ND:YAG laser
   E. Intensive Pulsed Light (IPL)

Q3. A 27-year-old female presents with fever, swelling, and redness in the left nasolabial fold two weeks after receiving dermal filler treatment. She reports feeling unwell and has been unable to contact the original treating clinician. On examination, there is a tense, fluctuant, erythematous area over the nasolabial fold. What is the most appropriate management?
   A. Prescribe oral antibiotics and monitor closely
   B. Inject hyaluronidase into the affected area
   C. Admit for intravenous antibiotics and incision and drainage
   D. Start topical corticosteroids to reduce inflammation
   E. Perform a bacterial culture and delay treatment until results are available

Q4. A 55-year-old woman presents with concerns about her low eyebrows and deep forehead wrinkles. She has prominent transverse forehead rhytids and noticeable brow asymmetry. Additionally, she reports thinning of her hair and is seeing another clinician for hair restoration treatments. Which of the following brow lift techniques is most appropriate for this patient?

 DOI: 10.1201/9781003609308-10

A. Direct brow lift
B. Midforehead brow lift
C. Coronal brow lift
D. Endoscopic brow lift
E. Trichophytic brow lift

Q5. A 67-year-old female presents with progressive drooping of her left upper eyelid, which has started to interfere with her vision. She has a history of cataract surgery in the same eye 10 years ago. Examination shows no significant eyebrow asymmetry, and her levator function is good. A phenylephrine test results in a marked improvement in eyelid position. What is the most appropriate surgical management for this patient?
A. Frontalis sling procedure
B. Levator advancement
C. Müller muscle-conjunctival resection
D. Fasanella-Servat procedure
E. Glasses with crutch attachment

Q6. A 42-year-old patient undergoes a lower blepharoplasty for the correction of puffy lower eyelids. Postoperatively, the patient reports diplopia, and examination reveals restricted gaze. Which of the following is the most likely cause?
A. Damage to the inferior rectus muscle
B. Excessive excision of lower lid tissue leading to scleral show
C. Damage to the inferior oblique muscle
D. Damage to the levator aponeurosis
E. Retrobulbar haemorrhage compressing orbital structures

Q7. During a parotidectomy, you encounter a patient with an aberrant facial nerve branch that loops superiorly before entering the parotid gland. What embryological variation is most likely responsible for this anomaly?
A. Duplication of the second pharyngeal arch
B. Persistence of the first pharyngeal arch structures
C. Altered migration of neural crest cells
D. Duplication of the facial nerve trunk
E. Persistent embryological connections to the hypoglossal nerve

Q8. A 55-year-old woman undergoes a deep-plane facelift. Which retaining ligament of the face is most critical to release to achieve significant midface elevation?
A. Buccal-maxillary ligament
B. Mandibular ligament
C. Orbital retaining ligament
D. Zygomatic retaining ligament
E. Masseteric cutaneous ligament

Q9. A 45-year-old male presents with difficulty in forming a full smile following trauma to the left side of his face. Examination reveals weakness in elevating the left upper lip and oral commissure. Which muscle is most likely affected?

A. Zygomaticus major
B. Levator labii superioris
C. Risorius
D. Buccinator
E. Orbicularis oris

Q10. A 45-year-old male undergoes excision of a forehead lesion, followed by primary closure. Which phase of wound healing is characterised by the significant increase in fibroblasts and deposition of collagen?
A. Inflammatory phase
B. Proliferative phase
C. Remodelling phase
D. Hemostasis phase
E. Maturation phase

Q11. A 45-year-old woman presents requesting treatment for glabellar frown lines. She has a history of myasthenia gravis, which is currently well controlled. Which of the following may exacerbate her underlying condition during treatment with botulinum toxin?
A. Competitive antagonism at postsynaptic acetylcholine receptors
B. Blockade of muscarinic receptors in sweat glands
C. Increased degradation of acetylcholine by acetylcholinesterase
D. Upregulation of nicotinic acetylcholine receptors
E. Inhibition of acetylcholine release at the neuromuscular junction

Q12. A 36-year-old male undergoes autologous fat grafting to correct facial asymmetry following trauma. Two months later, he develops swelling and induration at the graft site. What is the most likely explanation?
A. Graft rejection
B. Allergic reaction
C. Hematoma formation
D. Fat necrosis
E. Vascular compromise

Q13. A 42-year-old woman presents with delayed onset swelling, erythema, and pain at the site of a hyaluronic acid filler injection performed six months ago. What is the most likely cause?
A. Biofilm formation
B. Vascular occlusion
C. Type I hypersensitivity reaction
D. Subclinical infection
E. Migration of filler material

Q14. A 42-year-old male undergoes a laser procedure for deep skin resurfacing. The procedure uses a laser with a wavelength of 10,600 nm that vaporises tissue and coagulates vessels smaller than 0.5 mm in diameter. Which type of laser is most likely being used?
A. Pulsed dye laser
B. CO_2 laser

C. Potassium Titanyl Phosphate (KTP) laser
D. ND:YAG laser
E. Intensive Pulsed Light (IPL)

Q15. A 50-year-old female presents for treatment of fine wrinkles and dull skin texture. Which topical agent stimulates collagen production and improves skin quality?
A. Hyaluronic acid
B. Retinoic acid
C. Vitamin B6
D. Salicylic acid
E. Glycolic acid

Q16. A 38-year-old female undergoes a medium-depth chemical peel with trichloroacetic acid (TCA) for facial pigmentation. One week later, she presents with areas of erythema and dyspigmentation. What is the most likely cause of this complication?
A. Post-inflammatory hyperpigmentation
B. Chemical burn
C. Allergic reaction
D. Secondary bacterial infection
E. Reactivation of herpes simplex

Q17. A 30-year-old male presents with a dorsal hump and nasal deviation following trauma two years ago. During an open rhinoplasty procedure, what is the most important technique to ensure straightening of the deviated bony nasal pyramid?
A. Spreader graft placement
B. Lateral osteotomy
C. Medial osteotomy
D. Placement of columellar strut graft
E. Harvesting septal cartilage

Q18. A 42-year-old female presents with nasal obstruction and external deformity following septoplasty. Examination reveals a saddle nose deformity and nasal valve collapse. Which surgical intervention is most appropriate for both functional and aesthetic restoration?
A. Revision septoplasty with spreader grafts
B. Open rhinoplasty with septal extension graft
C. Closed rhinoplasty with dorsal hump reduction
D. Lateral osteotomy
E. Endoscopic sinus surgery

Q19. A 39-year-old man undergoes rhinoplasty. Six months later, he reports dissatisfaction with persistent tip deviation. Despite reassurance from three other surgeons that there is minimal deviation, he seeks revision surgery from you. Which of the following statements is correct?
A. Revision rhinoplasty should be offered immediately to address the patient's concerns
B. Patients dissatisfied with rhinoplasty outcomes commonly meet criteria for body dysmorphic disorder (BDD), which is common in the general population
C. Cognitive behavioural therapy (CBT) may be of benefit

D. Physical examination findings should always take precedence over psychological assessment in revision rhinoplasty cases
E. Body dysmorphic disorder symptoms are typically resolved by performing revision surgery

Q20. A 34-year-old woman presents with a "tombstone" appearance at the nasal tip following primary rhinoplasty. She is noted to have thin skin and low body mass. Which type of graft was most likely used in the original surgery?
A. Columellar strut graft
B. Shield graft
C. Alar batten graft
D. Dorsal onlay graft
E. Lateral crural strut graft

Q21. A 25-year-old male undergoing secondary rhinoplasty requires substantial graft material for structural support. Which of the following graft sources provides the most robust structural support for extensive nasal reconstruction?
A. Nasal septum cartilage
B. Conchal cartilage
C. Costochondral cartilage
D. Temporalis fascia
E. Auricular cartilage

Q22. A 58-year-old woman with dermatochalasis and visual field obstruction undergoes upper blepharoplasty. Postoperative lagophthalmos is noted. Which of the following was likely injured in the procedure resulting in this presentation?
A. Levator aponeurosis
B. Orbital septum
C. Preaponeurotic fat
D. Superior oblique muscle
E. Müller's muscle

Q23. A 28-year-old male presents with a retrusive chin. He undergoes a sliding genioplasty for correction. What is the most significant advantage of sliding genioplasty over alloplastic chin augmentation?
A. Improved soft tissue adherence
B. Reduced risk of infection
C. Ability to modify both projection and vertical height
D. Lower cost
E. Minimally invasive technique

Q24. A 52-year-old female undergoes an endoscopic brow lift for severe lateral brow ptosis. Which of the following structures must be released to achieve optimal elevation of the lateral brow?
A. Orbicularis retaining ligament
B. Superficial temporal fascia
C. Zygomatic retaining ligament
D. Corrugator supercilii muscle
E. Frontalis muscle

Q25. A 60-year-old male undergoes a neck lift for significant submental ptosis. During the procedure, the medial platysma is tightened. Which of the following complications is most likely to occur if excessive tension is applied during platysmaplasty?

A. Dysphagia
B. Sialocele formation
C. Marginal mandibular nerve injury
D. Hematoma
E. Asymmetrical neck contours

Q26. A 50-year-old male undergoes autologous fat grafting to correct midface volume loss following trauma. Which of the following factors most significantly determines long-term graft survival?

A. Volume of fat injected
B. Technique of fat harvesting
C. Use of tumescent solution
D. Depth of fat injection
E. Fat processing method

Q27. A 27-year-old transgender woman undergoes sliding genioplasty for facial feminisation. Which of the following modifications is most appropriate to achieve a feminine chin contour?

A. Reduction of chin height and narrowing
B. Advancement of the chin anteriorly
C. Vertical height augmentation
D. Bilateral augmentation with implants
E. Maintaining original chin contours

Q28. A 25-year-old transgender woman undergoes hairline advancement surgery. Which of the following complications is most likely if excessive tension is applied during the procedure?

A. Hair loss at the graft site
B. Infection of the graft site
C. Facial nerve injury
D. Hematoma formation
E. Hypertrophic scarring

Q29. A 12-year-old boy presents with bilateral prominent ear deformity and is scheduled for otoplasty. Which anatomical feature provides the primary structural support for ear shape?

A. Conchal cartilage
B. Helical rim
C. Antitragus
D. Auricular muscle
E. External acoustic meatus

Q30. 25-year-old male presents with a keloid scar on his left cheek following a laceration from a cycling accident six months ago. He is concerned about the appearance of the scar and asks about potential management options. Which of the following is the most appropriate initial treatment for this keloid?

A. Surgical excision of the keloid followed by immediate closure
B. Cryotherapy
C. Intralesional corticosteroid injections
D. Laser therapy
E. Topical silicone gel sheets

ANSWERS AND EXPLANATIONS

Q1. **Rhinophyma**

Answer: E. Surgical debulking

Explanation: Rhinophyma, a severe form of rosacea, is characterised by progressive thickening of nasal skin and a distorted, nodular nasal contour. This patient's significant nasal enlargement and psychological distress require a definitive intervention.

Surgical debulking is the most effective treatment for severe rhinophyma, as it removes the excess tissue and restores the natural nasal shape, directly addressing the patient's concerns.

- A. Topical metronidazole gel and B. oral isotretinoin are generally used to treat rosacea but are ineffective for managing the structural changes and tissue overgrowth in rhinophyma.
- C. Dermabrasion can improve skin texture but is insufficient for significant nasal thickening and distortion.
- D. Chemical peel may help with superficial skin changes but does not address the deep tissue hypertrophy characteristic of advanced rhinophyma.

For cases of severe rhinophyma with functional or psychological impacts, surgical debulking provides the most definitive and effective solution.

Q2. **Laser treatment**

Answer: C. Potassium Titanyl Phosphate (KTP) laser

Explanation: The Potassium Titanyl Phosphate (KTP) laser operates at a wavelength of 532 nm and targets oxyhaemoglobin, making it ideal for treating vascular lesions such as telangiectasia.

- A. CO_2 laser targets water and is used for excision, vaporisation, and deep skin resurfacing.
- B. Pulsed dye laser targets haemoglobin and melanin, but its wavelength (585 nm) is not as specific for oxyhaemoglobin.
- D. ND:YAG laser (1,064 nm) targets tissue proteins and is used for deep benign vascular lesions.
- E. IPL uses multiple wavelengths and is not a true laser.

Q3. **Dermal filler complications**

Answer: C. Admit for intravenous antibiotics and incision and drainage

Explanation: This presentation is consistent with an abscess following dermal filler injection. The correct management is incision and drainage combined with intravenous antibiotics. Delaying treatment in this scenario risks worsening the infection and potential complications, including midfacial or intracerebral involvement.

- A. Oral antibiotics alone are insufficient for managing this case as the patient is systemically unwell with a local collection needing drainage.
- B. Hyaluronidase is contraindicated in active infections, as it may spread the infection into adjacent tissues.
- D. Corticosteroids should not be used in the presence of infection, as they can exacerbate bacterial growth.
- E. While bacterial cultures are important, treatment should not be delayed in an actively infected abscess. Cultures should be obtained before initiating empiric antibiotic therapy.

Q4. **Brow lift**

Answer: B. Midforehead brow lift

Explanation: The midforehead brow lift is the most appropriate option for this patient because it uses the existing transverse rhytids to camouflage the incision and directly corrects the brow asymmetry. This technique is well-suited for patients with deep forehead wrinkles and avoids incisions in the hairline or scalp, which is ideal for someone with thinning hair.

- A. Direct brow lift: Suitable for patients with thick eyebrows or mild ptosis, but results in a visible scar, which is less ideal for this patient's needs.
- C. Coronal brow lift: Involves an incision across the scalp, which is contraindicated in this patient due to her thinning hair.
- D. Endoscopic brow lift: A minimally invasive option with hidden scars, but it is less effective in lifting heavy brows and correcting brow asymmetry.
- E. Trichophytic brow lift: Allows for forehead shortening and works well for patients with high hairlines, but its incisions near the hairline would be visible or problematic in patients with thinning hair.

Thus, the midforehead brow lift offers the best outcome for this patient's specific concerns and clinical findings.

Q5. **Upper lid ptosis**

Answer: C. Müller muscle-conjunctival resection

Explanation: This patient has aponeurotic ptosis, the most common cause of acquired ptosis, often associated with involutional changes or post-surgical changes, such as after cataract surgery. The positive phenylephrine test indicates that her eyelid responds well to stimulation of the sympathetic pathway, which makes the Müller muscle-conjunctival resection (internal levator advancement) the best option. This procedure elevates the ptotic lid without a skin incision, using a minimally invasive approach.

- A. Frontalis sling procedure: Used for severe ptosis, especially in cases of poor levator function, and typically involves suspending the eyelid from the frontalis muscle.
- B. Levator advancement: Suitable for ptosis with good levator function but without a significant response to the phenylephrine test.
- D. Fasanella-Servat procedure: Similar to the Mueller muscle-conjunctival resection but involves resection of tarsus and conjunctiva; not typically indicated in this case.
- E. Glasses with crutch attachment: Non-surgical option for patients who are not surgical candidates, but less effective and less cosmetic.

Q6. **Lower blepharoplasty complications**

Answer: C. Damage to the inferior oblique muscle

Explanation: The inferior oblique muscle, located between the medial and middle fat compartments of the lower eyelid, is at risk of injury during lower blepharoplasty. This muscle functions to elevate and abduct the eye, and damage can result in diplopia and specific gaze restrictions.

- A. Damage to the inferior rectus muscle: The inferior rectus controls downward gaze and is situated deeper within the orbit, forming the boundary of the intraconal space, making it less likely to be injured during lower blepharoplasty compared to the inferior oblique muscle.
- B. Excessive excision of lower lid tissue leading to scleral show: This complication causes cosmetic deformity and exposure keratopathy but does not typically result in diplopia or restricted gaze.
- D. Damage to the levator aponeurosis: This structure connects the levator palpebrae superioris muscle to the upper eyelid and is not involved in lower eyelid surgery, so it would not account for this presentation.
- E. Retrobulbar haemorrhage compressing orbital structures: This can lead to severe complications, including proptosis, vision loss, and pain.

Q7. **Embryology of facial nerve**

Answer: C. Altered migration of neural crest cells

Explanation: Neural crest cells contribute to the development of cranial nerves, including the facial nerve. Variations in their migration can result in aberrant branching patterns. The facial nerve supplies muscles of the second pharyngeal arch.

Q8. **Facelift anatomy**

Answer: D. Zygomatic retaining ligament

Explanation: The deep-plane facelift releases four key retaining ligaments in the face and neck, the zygomatic retaining, masseteric cutaneous, mandibular cutaneous, and cervical retaining ligaments. The zygomatic retaining ligament, resists skin sagging. Its release during deep-plane facelift allows repositioning and elevation of the midface soft tissue. Releasing the mandibular ligament is important to address marionette lines. Releasing the masseteric cutaneous ligaments is important to address the jawline.

Q9. **Mimetic muscles**

Answer: A. Zygomaticus major

Explanation: The zygomaticus major is primarily responsible for elevating the upper lip and pulling it supero-laterally to create a smile. Damage to this muscle or its nerve supply results in impaired smiling. Levator labii superioris assists in upper lip elevation but does not contribute significantly to lateral movement, so it is less important in smiling and laughing.

Q10. **Wound healing**

Answer: B. Proliferative phase

Explanation: Wound healing occurs in distinct phases:

1. Haemostasis phase (immediate): Platelets aggregate to form a clot and release cytokines like platelet-derived growth factor (PDGF) and transforming growth factor-beta (TGF-β), initiating the healing cascade.
2. Inflammatory phase (0–3 days): Neutrophils and macrophages infiltrate the wound to phagocytose debris and pathogens. Pro-inflammatory cytokines, such as interleukin-1 (IL-1) and tumour necrosis factor-alpha (TNF-α), recruit additional immune cells.
3. Proliferative phase (4–21 days): Fibroblasts proliferate and produce collagen type III. Angiogenesis occurs, driven by vascular endothelial growth factor (VEGF). Granulation tissue forms, providing a framework for epithelialisation.
4. Remodelling/maturation phase (21 days–1 year): Collagen type III is replaced by collagen type I. The wound achieves tensile strength, and excess capillaries regress. Scar tissue forms, often with a decrease in overall skin elasticity.

Q11. **Botulinum toxin**

Answer: E. Inhibition of acetylcholine release at the neuromuscular junction

Explanation: Botulinum toxin acts by inhibiting acetylcholine release at the neuromuscular junction, which can exacerbate myasthenia gravis, a condition characterised by impaired neuromuscular transmission.

Q12. **Fat grafting**

Answer: D. Fat necrosis

Explanation: Fat necrosis is a known complication of autologous fat grafting, occurring due to inadequate revascularisation of the grafted fat. This results in firm, non-tender nodules. Graft rejection is not relevant, as autologous tissue is used, and vascular compromise typically presents acutely.

Q13. **Dermal filler complications**

Answer: A. Biofilm formation

Explanation: Biofilm formation is a delayed complication of dermal fillers, resulting from bacterial colonisation around the filler material. It can present with chronic inflammation and swelling, requiring treatment with antibiotics and, in some cases, hyaluronidase.

Q14. **Laser treatment**

Answer: B. CO_2 laser

Explanation: The CO_2 laser operates at a wavelength of 10,600 nm and targets water as its chromophore. It is used for excision, vaporisation, and deep skin resurfacing, offering coagulation of vessels smaller than 0.5 mm in diameter.

- A. Pulsed dye laser targets haemoglobin and melanin, not water, and operates at 585 nm.
- C. KTP laser operates at 532 nm and targets oxyhaemoglobin, not used for resurfacing.
- D. ND:YAG laser targets tissue proteins at 1,064 nm and is used for vascular lesions, not deep resurfacing.
- E. IPL is not a laser and uses multiple wavelengths for general skin treatments like scars or wrinkles.

Q15. **Retinoic acid**

Answer: B. Retinoic acid

Explanation: Retinoic acid stimulates collagen production and accelerates epidermal turnover, improving wrinkles and skin texture. Hyaluronic acid hydrates the skin but does not stimulate collagen production, while glycolic acid and salicylic acid provide chemical exfoliation. Vitamin B6 is pyridoxine. Deficiency can lead to dermatitis and chelitis. Vitamin C is a cofactor for the enzymes prolyl hydroxylase and lysyl hydroxylase, which are essential for collagen biosynthesis. It also stabilises the tertiary structure of collagen.

Q16. **Chemical peel**

Answer: A. Post-inflammatory hyperpigmentation

Explanation: Post-inflammatory hyperpigmentation is a common complication of medium-depth chemical peels, particularly in individuals with darker skin tones. Proper patient selection and pre-treatment with depigmenting agents can reduce this risk. Reactivation of herpes simplex can occur and many advocate prophylactic acyclovir if patients have a strong history of recurrent episodes.

Q17. **Open rhinoplasty**

Answer: B. Lateral osteotomy

Explanation: Lateral osteotomies are critical for mobilising and realigning the bony nasal pyramid in cases of deviation. Spreader grafts address internal valve narrowing but do not correct bony deformities.

Q18. **Open rhinoplasty**

Answer: B. Open rhinoplasty with septal extension graft

Explanation: A septal extension graft restores structural support to the nasal tip and midline, addressing both saddle deformity and nasal valve collapse. Revision septoplasty alone would not adequately restore external deformities.

Q19. **Psychological component of facial aesthetics**

Answer: C. Cognitive behavioural therapy (CBT) may be of benefit for patients with disproportionate distress over minor cosmetic irregularities

Explanation: Patients seeking revision rhinoplasty often have underlying psychological factors, including concerns disproportionate to objective findings. CBT is evidence-based and effective for managing patients with distress over perceived cosmetic flaws, particularly those with features suggestive of BDD. While BDD is not common in the general population, it is overrepresented among patients undergoing cosmetic procedures. Immediate revision surgery is not recommended, as it may reinforce psychological distress rather than alleviate it. Physical findings should be evaluated alongside psychological health. Surgery rarely resolves BDD symptoms, which often persist regardless of cosmetic outcomes.

Q20. **Complications of rhinoplasty**

Answer: B. Shield graft

Explanation: Shield grafts are placed over the medial crura to enhance nasal tip projection and definition. In patients with thin skin, these grafts can create a visible "tombstone" appearance due to insufficient tissue coverage. This is less of an issue in patients with thicker skin. Proper bevelling and edge refinement during graft placement can help minimise visibility.

Q21. **Secondary rhinoplasty**

Answer: C. Costochondral cartilage

Explanation: Costochondral cartilage provides a strong and durable graft for structural support in nasal reconstruction. Septal and conchal cartilage are less robust and limited in volume.

Q22. **Upper blepharoplasty**

Answer: A. Levator aponeurosis

Explanation: Preservation of the levator aponeurosis is essential to maintain eyelid function and prevent postoperative lagophthalmos/ptosis. Excessive resection of this structure may result in impaired eyelid closure/incompetence. Müller's muscle is a smooth muscle on the underside of the levator aponeurosis with sympathetic innervation. Although it contributes to elevation of the upper lid, it has less of a contribution compared to levator palpebrae superioris (skeletal muscle under voluntary control).

Q23. **Genioplasty**

Answer: C. Ability to modify both projection and vertical height

Explanation: Sliding genioplasty allows precise modification of chin projection and vertical height, which is not possible with alloplastic implants. Infection risk is also lower compared to implants, but this is not the primary advantage.

Q24. **Brow lift**

Answer: A. Orbicularis retaining ligament

Explanation: Releasing the orbicularis retaining ligament allows for lateral brow elevation and smooth repositioning of the skin. The corrugator supercilii muscle is typically addressed to reduce vertical glabellar lines but does not significantly affect lateral brow ptosis.

Q25. **Neck lift complications**

Answer: A. Dysphagia

Explanation: Excessive tension during medial platysmaplasty can restrict the movement of the underlying hyoid musculature, leading to dysphagia. Careful technique and tension adjustment can mitigate this risk.

Q26. **Fat grafting**

Answer: B. Technique of fat harvesting

Explanation: Fat graft survival depends primarily on the preservation of intact mature adipocytes and mesenchymal stem cells in the stromal component. The technique of fat harvesting, including low-pressure suction and minimal trauma to adipocytes, is critical for graft survival. Fat processing methods are important to remove debris from traumatic adipocyte rupture erythrocytes, etc. It is also important for long-term fat graft survival but secondary to atraumatic harvesting with appropriate techniques.

Q27. **Genioplasty**

Answer: A. Reduction of chin height and narrowing

Explanation: Feminine chin contours typically involve a narrower and less prominent chin with reduced vertical height. This contrasts with a more square and robust chin in masculine features.

Q28. **Hairline advancement**

Answer: A. Hair loss at the graft site

Explanation: Excessive tension during hairline advancement can compromise the blood supply to the frontal scalp, resulting in hair loss at the graft site. Proper tension management reduces this risk.

Q29. **Otoplasty**

Answer: A. Conchal cartilage

Explanation: Conchal cartilage forms the core structural support for the auricle and determines the ear's overall shape. In otoplasty, modifications to the conchal cartilage are key to achieving an aesthetically pleasing result.

Q30. **Keloid scarring**

Answer: C. Intralesional corticosteroid injections, which help to reduce inflammation and collagen production, leading to scar softening and flattening.

Explanation: The most effective initial treatment for keloid scars is typically intralesional corticosteroid injections. These injections reduce collagen synthesis, inflammation, and vascularity within the keloid, leading to flattening, softening, and a reduction in size over time. Intralesional steroids such as triamcinolone acetonide are commonly used for this purpose. This approach is non-invasive and is often the first-line therapy for keloids, especially on visible areas like the face. Surgical excision carries a high risk of recurrence, particularly for facial keloids. It's generally avoided. Laser therapy, while useful for improving pigmentation and texture in some scars, has limited efficacy in reducing the size and volume of keloids. Topical silicone gel sheets are commonly used for scar prevention and can be effective in improving the appearance of scars in the early stages but often ineffective for established keloids.

10 Dentoalveolar

QUESTIONS

Q1. A 22-year-old patient presents with localised pain, swelling, and limited mouth opening associated with a partially erupted lower third molar. This is their first episode, and there are no signs of systemic infection. What is the most appropriate management?

A. Immediate extraction of the lower third molar
B. Prescribe systemic antibiotics alone
C. Irrigation and oral hygiene instruction
D. Rebook for surgical removal of the tooth
E. Prescribe topical antiseptic mouthwash

Q2. A 38-year-old male requires a bone graft to augment a localised defect in the anterior maxilla. Harvesting from the mandible is planned. Which of the following sites provides the largest quantity of cancellous bone while minimising donor site morbidity?

A. Symphysis of the mandible
B. Lingual plate of the ramus
C. Buccal shelf of the mandible
D. External oblique ridge
E. Coronoid process

Q3. A 55-year-old patient presents with a draining oral-cutaneous fistula originating from a non-vital mandibular molar. What is the most appropriate next step in management?

A. Antibiotics and regular follow-up
B. Immediate surgical closure of the fistula
C. Extraction of the involved tooth
D. Biopsy of the fistula tract
E. Marsupialisation of the fistula tract

Q4. A 60-year-old patient presents with a persistent oral-antral fistula (OAF) 6 months after dental extraction. The patient reports intermittent nasal regurgitation and a history of sinusitis. What is the most appropriate management?

A. Observation and nasal irrigation
B. Closure with a buccal fat pad flap
C. Endoscopic sinus surgery followed by primary closure
D. Excision of fistulous tract and closure with buccal advancement flap
E. Antibiotics and follow-up in three months

DOI: 10.1201/9781003609308-11

Q5. A 45-year-old patient undergoes extraction of the upper first molar. You suspect there may be a very small oro-antral communication. There is no evidence of infection. What is the most appropriate immediate management?
A. Prescribe antibiotics and observe
B. Immediate closure with a buccal advancement flap
C. Pack the socket with resorbable collagen and advise sinus precautions
D. Perform Caldwell-Luc surgery for sinus obliteration
E. Refer for secondary closure in six weeks

Q6. A 10-year-old child presents after trauma to the maxillary central incisors. Examination reveals that one tooth is mobile and displaced but still within the socket, while the adjacent tooth is fractured at the enamel-dentin junction without pulp exposure. How should the mobile tooth be managed?
A. Rigid splinting for four weeks with orthodontic follow-up
B. Immediate extraction
C. Observation and soft diet with no intervention
D. Repositioning and flexible splinting for two weeks
E. Repositioning and flexible splinting for four weeks

Q7. A 12-year-old child presents three days after trauma to the maxillary central incisors. Examination reveals that the UL1 is mobile and displaced palatally, while the UR1 has suffered a complicated crown fracture with pulp exposure. What is the most appropriate management option for UR1?
A. Immediate extraction of the tooth
B. Indirect pulp capping with calcium hydroxide
C. Partial pulpotomy with calcium hydroxide or MTA
D. Root canal treatment with gutta-percha obturation
E. Watchful waiting with follow-up in six months

Q8. A 45-year-old patient is undergoing a prolonged complex dentoalveolar surgery under local anaesthesia. Which of the following best explains the pharmacodynamic properties that make bupivacaine suitable for such a procedure?
A. Low lipid solubility
B. High protein binding
C. Low ionisation and high diffusion through nerve membranes
D. High vasodilation leading to increased systemic absorption
E. Short half-life and low systemic toxicity

Q9. A 32-year-old patient presents with a deeply impacted mandibular third molar associated with the inferior alveolar nerve. A coronectomy is planned to minimise nerve injury. Which of the following would contraindicate the procedure?
A. Absence of infection around the impacted tooth
B. Periodontal disease
C. Radiographic proximity of the roots to the inferior alveolar nerve
D. Crown covered entirely by dense bone
E. Early occlusal caries confined to enamel

Q10. A 35-year-old patient presents with altered sensation over the lower lip and chin following mandibular third molar extraction. Examination reveals no response to

light touch, but nerve conduction studies show slowed conduction. According to Seddon's classification, how should this injury be classified?
A. Neuropraxia
B. Axonotmesis
C. Neurotmesis
D. Neuroma
E. Wallerian degeneration

Q11. A 29-year-old male presents with a painless swelling in the left mandibular parasymphysis. Imaging reveals a large, well-defined radiolucency with thinning of the cortical bone and displacement of the mental nerve, which appears to run through the lesion. Incisional biopsy shows non-keratinised stratified squamous epithelium with mucous cells with no dysplasia. Which of the following is the most appropriate initial management?
A. Enucleation with primary closure
B. Marsupialization and decompression
C. Segmental resection of the mandible with reconstruction
D. Observation with periodic radiographic monitoring
E. Surgical curettage with chemical cauterisation

Q12. During the surgical extraction of an upper left third molar, the tooth is inadvertently displaced posteriorly. Into which anatomical space is the tooth most likely displaced?
A. Maxillary sinus
B. Buccal space
C. Infratemporal fossa
D. Retropharyngeal space
E. Pterygopalatine fossa

Q13. A 34-year-old male presents with swelling in the posterior mandible. Panoramic radiography reveals a well-defined, unilocular radiolucency extending from the mandibular first molar to the angle of the mandible. The lesion has caused thinning of the cortical bone but no perforation or root resorption. Histological analysis from an incisional biopsy confirms the lesion to be lined by keratinised epithelium. Which of the following is the most appropriate management?
A. Marsupialization followed by delayed enucleation
B. Wide local excision with bone grafting
C. Enucleation with or without adjunctive treatment
D. Observation with regular radiographic follow-up
E. Segmental resection of the mandible

Q14. A patient is undergoing a sinus lift procedure to facilitate placement of a dental implant in the posterior maxilla. What is the most important factor to ensure the success of the procedure?
A. Adequate bone height before sinus lift
B. Integrity of the Schneiderian membrane
C. The length of the dental implant
D. Use of autologous bone grafts
E. Width of alveolar bone before sinus lift

Q15. During the surgical extraction of an impacted upper right third molar (UR8), a palatal tear is noted with brisk arterial bleeding from the palate. The patient is on apixaban for AF. Which of the following is the most likely to achieve successful haemostasis?

A. Pack the area with oxidised cellulose and apply firm pressure
B. Identify and ligate the greater palatine artery
C. Pack the maxillary sinus with hemostatic material via the socket
D. Elevate the head and provide systemic tranexamic acid
E. Perform immediate exploration of the pterygopalatine fossa

Q16. A 35-year-old male presents with swelling and a radiolucent lesion in the posterior mandible associated with an unerupted third molar. Histopathology reveals reduced enamel epithelium lining the cyst. What is the most likely diagnosis?

A. Odontogenic keratocyst
B. Dentigerous cyst
C. Ameloblastoma
D. Lateral periodontal cyst
E. Radicular cyst

Q17. A 12-year-old child presents with multiple unerupted teeth, and radiographs reveal numerous unerupted supernumerary teeth throughout the maxilla and mandible. Which congenital syndrome is most likely associated with this presentation?

A. Treacher Collins syndrome
B. Cleidocranial dysplasia
C. Crouzon syndrome
D. Apert syndrome
E. Gorlin syndrome

Q18. A 7-year-old boy presents with delayed dental eruption and complaints of difficulty chewing. Clinical examination reveals peg-shaped incisors and multiple missing teeth. His mother mentions he has thin, brittle hair and often struggles with overheating during summer. Which of the following is the most likely diagnosis?

A. Amelogenesis imperfecta
B. Hypohidrotic ectodermal dysplasia
C. Cleidocranial dysplasia
D. Rickets
E. Congenital hypothyroidism

Q19. A 68-year-old patient with atrial fibrillation and poorly controlled diabetes is scheduled for extraction of LL8 and UL8 under local anaesthesia. The LL8 is mesially impacted. The patient is on apixaban for anticoagulation. What is the most appropriate perioperative management plan regarding apixaban?

A. Continue apixaban without interruption.
B. Stop apixaban 36 hours before the procedure and restart 24 hours later.
C. Stop apixaban 24 hours before the procedure and restart the evening dose after 6 hours.

D. Omit the morning dose of apixaban on the day of the procedure and restart six hours post-procedure.
E. Switch to low-molecular-weight heparin for anticoagulation 48 hours prior to the procedure.

Q20. A 67-year-old male presents with exposed necrotic bone in the posterior mandible three months after radiation therapy for oropharyngeal cancer. He reports pain and swelling in the area, with purulent discharge. Imaging reveals sequestrum formation but no evidence of pathological fractures, fistulas, or skin involvement. Which of the following is correct?
A. The patient has Grade 0 ORN (modified Glanzmann and Graetz), requiring only observation.
B. The patient has Grade 2 ORN (modified Glanzmann and Graetz), requiring management of infection and potential debridement.
C. The patient has Stage I ORN (Notani), requiring no intervention.
D. The patient has Stage II ORN (Notani), requiring surgical resection.
E. The patient has Grade 3 ORN (modified Glanzmann and Graetz), requiring surgical resection.

Q21. A 63-year-old male presents with exposed necrotic bone in the posterior mandible six months after completing radiation therapy for oropharyngeal cancer. The affected area shows no signs of healing despite conservative management. Which of the following best describes the current understanding of the pathophysiology of osteoradionecrosis of the jaws (ORN)?
A. ORN is caused by trauma-induced infection in irradiated tissues.
B. ORN results from hypoxia, hypovascularity, and hypocellularity in irradiated bone.
C. ORN has to have been present for at least six weeks to meet the definition.
D. ORN develops from progressive destruction of the bone matrix by reactive oxygen species and microvascular necrosis.
E. ORN occurs exclusively due to radiation-induced bacterial overgrowth in the jaw.

Q22. A 67-year-old female with a history of head and neck radiotherapy for nasopharyngeal carcinoma presents with mandibular osteoradionecrosis (ORN). She has exposed necrotic bone in the mandible despite initial conservative measures. Which of the following statements about the treatment modalities for ORN is correct?
A. Surgical resection with microvascular reconstruction is the first-line treatment for advanced grades of ORN.
B. Curettage and removal of sequestrum is of benefit for early ORN of the jaw.
C. Pentoxifylline in the PENTO regimen primarily promotes osteoblast activity for bone regeneration.
D. Hyperbaric oxygen therapy has consistent high-level evidence supporting its use for ORN.
E. Pharmacological approaches, including the PENTO regimen, are only effective for ORN with pathological fractures.

Q23. A 29-year-old patient presents with a horizontally impacted lower left third molar. Cone beam computed tomography (CBCT) confirms a high risk of inferior dental nerve (IDN) injury if the tooth is extracted. The tooth is asymptomatic, and the pulp is vital. The clinician considers coronectomy. Which of the following statements is correct?

A. Coronectomy should be discussed for any lower third molar extraction
B. Root migration after coronectomy is uncommon and occurs in less than 5% of cases.
C. Coronectomy is contraindicated in mandibular third molars with a vital pulp.
D. Persistent apical infection is a potential complication that may necessitate reoperation after coronectomy.
E. CBCT assessment is not recommended in cases where coronectomy is planned.

Q24. A 45-year-old male presents with a chronic orocutaneous infection secondary to significant facial trauma sustained three months ago. On delayed presentation, he undergoes wound debridement, and cultures reveal an extended-spectrum beta-lactamase (ESBL)-producing organism. Which of the following is the most appropriate antibiotic regimen?

A. Amoxicillin-clavulanic acid
B. Ceftriaxone
C. Meropenem
D. Vancomycin
E. Piperacillin-tazobactam

Q25. A 42-year-old female presents with a severe headache, fever, periorbital swelling, and confusion. On examination, there is an obvious canine space collection as well as proptosis, ophthalmoplegia, and reduced vision in the left eye. She has a history of a long-standing, untreated dental infection associated with the upper left canine (UL3). Which of the following statements is true?

A. Imaging is not required, as diagnosis is purely clinical.
B. Anticoagulation is contraindicated due to the risk of bleeding.
C. Surgical drainage of the thrombus is required in all cases.
D. Dental infection is the most common cause of this presentation.
E. Mortality rate may be as high as 30%.

Q26. A 55-year-old male presents to his dentist with concerns about discomfort and bleeding around a dental implant placed six months ago. On examination, there is redness and swelling of the peri-implant mucosa, bleeding on gentle probing (0.2 N), and a probing depth of 4 mm. Radiographs show no marginal bone loss. Which of the following statements is true?

A. Peri-implant mucositis is characterised by inflammation and progressive bone loss surrounding the implant.
B. Peri-implantitis lesions are smaller than peri-implant mucositis lesions and contain fewer B-cells.
C. Peri-implant mucositis can be diagnosed based on the presence of inflammation without marginal bone loss.
D. A probing depth ≥6 mm is required to confirm the diagnosis of peri-implant mucositis.
E. Histological studies of peri-implant mucositis reveal a higher density of osteoclast-activating cytokines compared to peri-implantitis lesions.

Q27. A 47-year-old patient presents with symptomatic periradicular disease in a tooth with a post-retained crown restoration. Previous root canal treatment was performed to guideline standards, but the symptoms persist. The dentist is considering apicectomy. Which of the following statements is correct?

A. Apicectomy is indicated when there is a well-root-filled tooth with persistent periradicular disease and a high risk of root fracture from post removal.
B. Apicectomy is primarily indicated when there is no alternative option for restoring the tooth.
C. A poor coronal seal does not affect the outcome of an apicectomy if the root end is adequately resected.
D. Apicectomy is contraindicated in cases of symptomatic periradicular disease with persistent exudation into the root canal despite chemo-mechanical debridement.
E. The need for histopathological examination of periradicular tissues is not a valid indication for apicectomy.

Q28. A 38-year-old patient is undergoing an apicectomy for persistent periradicular disease associated with a previously root-filled molar. The surgeon is planning the procedure. Which of the following statements is correct?

A. A semilunar flap is the best choice for minimising scarring and providing adequate surgical access.
B. Osteotomies greater than 10 mm in diameter are preferred to improve visualisation of the root apex and apical tissues.
C. Root-end resection should be bevelled to minimise exposed dentinal tubules and reduce the risk of leakage.
D. Root-end preparation should be performed using ultrasonic retrotips to facilitate proper sealing with a root-end filling material.
E. Amalgam is the recommended material for root-end filling due to its superior biocompatibility and clinical outcomes.

Q29. A 30-year-old patient returns to your clinic two weeks after extraction of their lower left third molar (LL8). They complain of persistent numbness in their lower lip and chin on the left side. Examination reveals reduced sensation in the distribution of the inferior alveolar nerve but no other significant findings. What is the most appropriate management?

A. Reassure the patient and review again in six months.
B. Immediately refer the patient for surgical decompression of the inferior alveolar nerve.
C. Prescribe a course of corticosteroids to reduce inflammation around the nerve.
D. Refer the patient to a specialist centre if there is no improvement in sensation by three months post-injury.
E. Refer the patient to a specialist centre if there is no improvement in sensation by two months post-injury.

Q30. A 55-year-old male patient presents to the dental clinic with significant intraoral bleeding following a routine dental extraction. Which of the following statements is true regarding the medications and conditions that affect bleeding and coagulation?

A. Warfarin increases the activity of vitamin K-dependent clotting factors II, VII, IX, and X.
B. Tranexamic acid promotes fibrinolysis by increasing plasminogen activation to plasmin.
C. Aspirin irreversibly inhibits thromboxane A2, a key molecule in platelet aggregation.
D. Haemophilia A and B are characterised by elevated clotting factor levels VIII and IX, leading to an increased risk of bleeding.
E. Clopidogrel has no effect on platelet aggregation and is safe to use during surgical procedures involving bleeding risk.

Q31. A 34-year-old patient with a vital lower right third molar presents for evaluation. Cone beam computed tomography (CBCT) reveals the tooth is in close proximity to the inferior dental nerve (IDN), placing it at high risk for nerve injury during extraction. The clinician opts for coronectomy. Which of the following is true regarding coronectomy?
A. Coronectomy is contraindicated for mandibular third molars with a high risk of IDN injury.
B. The success rate of coronectomy is consistently above 95% in all studies.
C. Root migration after coronectomy may occur, but it is not always clinically significant.
D. Coronectomy eliminates the need for further monitoring or potential reoperation.
E. Vital pulp status is not a factor when considering coronectomy.

Q32. A 45-year-old male presents with a firm, non-tender swelling along the angle of his jaw that has gradually increased in size over the past few weeks. He reports a recent history of dental extraction. Examination reveals multiple draining sinus tracts discharging thick pus containing yellow granules. There is no significant lymphadenopathy. What is the most appropriate management option?
A. Oral co-amoxiclav for seven to ten days
B. IV co-amoxiclav for two weeks
C. IV ceftriaxone for four weeks followed by six weeks of doxycycline
D. IV meropenem for two weeks followed by six months of clarithromycin
E. IV co-amoxiclav for four weeks followed by six months of amoxicillin

ANSWERS AND EXPLANATIONS

Q1. **Pericoronitis**

Answer: C. Irrigation and oral hygiene instruction

Explanation: For a first episode of localised pericoronitis, management involves conservative measures such as irrigation of the operculum, oral hygiene instruction, and analgesics. Systemic antibiotics are only indicated for signs of systemic involvement or abscess. Immediate extraction is not recommended during the acute phase. Removal is reserved for recurrent episodes of pericoronitis rather than a single episode. Antiseptic mouthwash may be adjunctive but is not sufficient as the primary management.

Q2. **Autologous bone harvesting**

Answer: A. Symphysis of the mandible

Explanation: The symphysis of the mandible provides a significant quantity of cancellous bone for grafting and is easily accessible with minimal morbidity, although care must be taken to avoid damage to the mental nerves and incisive vessels. The external oblique ridge provides predominantly cortical bone. The buccal shelf and lingual plate of the ramus are less commonly used due to limited access and risk to adjacent structures. The coronoid process offers limited graft material.

Q3. **Dentoalveolar infection**

Answer: C. Extraction of the involved tooth

Explanation: Removal of the causative tooth may allow the fistula to heal spontaneously and prevents progression. Biopsy is only indicated if malignancy is suspected but can be performed concurrently when the tooth is extracted. Surgical closure of the fistula can be delayed until the infection is controlled.

Q4. **Oral-antral fistula**

Answer: D. Excision of fistulous tract and closure with buccal advancement flap

Explanation: OAFs require surgical closure due to their persistent communication between the oral cavity and maxillary sinus. Excision of the fistulous tract ensures complete removal of granulation tissue, and a buccal advancement flap provides a reliable closure.

Q5. **Oral-antral communication**

Answer: C. Pack the socket with resorbable collagen and advise sinus precautions

Explanation: Small oral-antral communications (≤5 mm) can be managed conservatively by packing the socket with resorbable material and advising the patient on sinus precautions, such as avoiding nose-blowing and sneezing with a closed mouth. Buccal advancement flaps are reserved for larger defects or those persisting beyond 48–72 hours. Antibiotics may be considered to prevent sinus infection but are not the definitive management.

Q6. **Dentoalveolar trauma**

Answer: E. Repositioning and splinting for four weeks

Explanation: The mobile tooth is consistent with lateral luxation, characterised by displacement with alveolar bone injury. As a result, longer flexible splinting time of four weeks is recommended. A two-week flexible splint is used for extrusions and some avulsion injuries (depending on extra-oral dry time). Rigid splinting not recommended as increased likelihood of ankylosis or external resorption.

Q7. **Dentoalveolar trauma**

Answer: C. Partial pulpotomy with calcium hydroxide or MTA

Explanation: A complicated crown fracture with pulp exposure in a young permanent tooth requires vital pulp therapy to preserve pulp vitality and allow continued root development. A partial pulpotomy using calcium hydroxide or mineral trioxide aggregate (MTA) is the treatment of choice, as it removes the superficial inflamed pulp while preserving the deeper healthy pulp. Immediate extraction is not necessary, as the tooth can be salvaged. Indirect pulp capping is only suitable for cases without pulp exposure. Root canal treatment is premature in a young tooth with an open apex and should only be considered if pulp necrosis occurs. Watchful waiting is inappropriate, as untreated pulp exposure leads to infection and necrosis.

Q8. **Pharmacology of local anaesthetic**

Answer: B. High protein binding

Explanation: Bupivacaine has a long duration of action (and half-life) due to its high protein binding, which prolongs its retention at the site of action and delays systemic absorption. Bupivacaine has high lipid solubility but slower onset compared to agents like lidocaine.

Q9. **Coronectomy**

Answer: E. Periodontal disease

Explanation: Coronectomy is contraindicated in cases where the retained roots may become a future source of infection or complications. Periodontal disease is a contraindication because it can lead to progressive bone loss, root exposure, and potential infection, increasing the risk of needing a secondary procedure. Other contraindications include root mobility, as unstable roots may migrate and require later removal, and periapical pathology or active infection involving the roots, which could lead to persistent infection. In contrast, radiographic proximity of the roots to the inferior alveolar nerve is an indication for coronectomy rather than a contraindication, as the procedure is specifically designed to prevent nerve injury in such cases. Dense bone completely covering the crown does not preclude coronectomy, though it may make access more challenging. Early occlusal caries confined to enamel is not a contraindication unless it extends to the retained roots.

Q10. **Nerve injury**

Answer: A. Neuropraxia

Explanation: Axonotmesis involves disruption of axonal continuity with intact nerve sheaths, leading to sensory loss but preserving the potential for regeneration. Neuropraxia involves transient conduction block without structural damage as indicated here by the preserved axonal continuity on nerve conduction study. Neurotmesis is complete nerve disruption, typically requiring surgical repair.

Q11. **Management of odontogenic cysts**

Answer: B. Marsupialization and decompression

Explanation: Marsupialization is the preferred initial management for large cysts involving vital structures (in this case the mental nerve), as it decompresses the lesion, reduces pressure, and preserves anatomy. Once the lesion is reduced in size, enucleation may be performed.

Q12. **Fascial spaces of the head and neck**

Answer: C. Infratemporal fossa

Explanation: Displacement of teeth during extraction may be a result of inappropriate force or poor technique. Removal of displaced teeth should be approached with preoperative imaging and good access. This helps to minimise complications, such as significant haemorrhage, due to injury to important anatomical structures in the infratemporal fossa.

Q13. **Management of odontogenic cysts**

Answer: C. Enucleation with or without adjunctive treatment

Explanation: Enucleation is the standard management for keratinised cystic lesions such as odontogenic keratocysts, provided the lesion is well-defined and does not extensively invade surrounding structures. Enucleation involves complete removal of the cyst lining, minimising the risk of recurrence. Adjunctive treatments such as chemical cauterisation (e.g., Carnoy's solution) or cryotherapy may be considered to further reduce recurrence rates. Marsupialization (A) is an alternative for large cysts when immediate enucleation risks damage to adjacent structures.

Q14. **Bone augmentation procedures**

Answer: B. Integrity of the Schneiderian membrane

Explanation: The integrity of the Schneiderian membrane (sinus lining) is critical for a successful sinus lift and implant placement. Perforations result in direct communication between the graft and the sinus cavity, exposing the graft to the sinus's microbial flora which can lead to graft failure or sinus complications. While bone height and width, implant length, graft type, and patient factors are important, maintaining membrane integrity is paramount for procedural success.

Q15. **Complications of dental extractions**

Answer: B. Identify and ligate the greater palatine artery

Explanation: Brisk arterial bleeding from the palate during maxillary third molar extraction is likely due to injury to the greater palatine artery, which courses anteriorly from the greater palatine foramen. Direct ligation or cauterisation of the artery at the site of bleeding is the most definitive management. Packing with hemostatic material is often a sensible first step but may be insufficient for active arterial bleeding. Maxillary sinus packing is unrelated to palatal bleeding. Systemic tranexamic acid addresses generalised bleeding tendencies but alone is unlikely to be effective for localised arterial haemorrhage. Exploration of the pterygopalatine fossa is overly invasive and not required for isolated palatal artery injury.

Q16. **Odontogenic cysts**

Answer: B. Dentigerous cyst

Explanation: Dentigerous cysts are odontogenic cysts associated with the crown of an unerupted tooth. They result from the accumulation of fluid between the reduced enamel epithelium and the tooth, typically in the mandibular third molar region.

Q17. **Syndromes of the head and neck**

Answer: B. Cleidocranial dysplasia

Explanation: Cleidocranial dysplasia is characterised by multiple unerupted supernumerary teeth, delayed eruption of permanent teeth, and skeletal abnormalities, such as partial or absent clavicles. This syndrome results from mutations in the RUNX2 gene.

Q18. **Syndromes of the head and neck**

Answer: B. Hypohidrotic ectodermal dysplasia

Explanation: The combination of dental anomalies (peg-shaped teeth and hypodontia), brittle hair, and reduced sweating strongly suggests hypohidrotic ectodermal dysplasia. This condition arises from abnormalities in ectodermal structures and is often associated with overheating due to defective sweat glands.

Q19. **Perioperative management for dentoalveolar surgery**

Answer: D. Omit the morning dose of apixaban on the day of the procedure and restart 6 hours post-procedure.

Explanation: Dental extractions, including the removal of up to three teeth or procedures with higher bleeding risks, can generally be performed safely with minor adjustments to apixaban. The optimal approach in this scenario is to omit the morning dose of apixaban to reduce intraoperative bleeding risk while ensuring that the anticoagulation is not unduly interrupted. Restarting apixaban six hours after the procedure ensures adequate hemostasis before resuming anticoagulation. Stopping apixaban 24–36 hours prior to the procedure is unnecessary for a procedure with manageable bleeding risk and increases the risk of thromboembolism. Switching to low-molecular-weight heparin is not indicated for this type of procedure (24).

Q20. **Osteoradionecrosis classification**

Answer: B. The patient has Grade 2 ORN (modified Glanzmann and Graetz), requiring management of infection and potential debridement.

Explanation: The modified Glanzmann and Graetz Grading system defines Grade 2 ORN as exposed necrotic bone with infection or sequestrum formation, which matches this patient's symptoms of exposed bone, purulent discharge, and sequestrum on imaging. This condition requires management of infection and possible debridement to prevent progression. Grade 3 ORN (modified Glanzmann and Graetz) involves pathological fractures or surgical resection, neither of which applies to this case.

Q21. **Osteoradionecrosis pathophysiology**

Answer: D. ORNJ develops from progressive destruction of the bone matrix by reactive oxygen species and microvascular necrosis.

Explanation: ORN of the jaws is defined as an area of devitalised, exposed bone resulting from head and neck radiation therapy, which fails to heal after three to six months without local signs of neoplastic disease. The current understanding of ORN is best explained by the RIF (radiation-induced fibrosis) theory, proposed by Delanian and Lefaix. This theory highlights that ORNJ results from the accumulation of reactive oxygen species (ROS) and radiation-induced damage to endothelial cells and fibroblasts. These processes lead to microvascular necrosis, impaired tissue repair, and altered collagen metabolism, causing progressive bone matrix destruction.

While earlier theories, such as Meyer's theory, focused on trauma-induced infection, or Marx's 3H hypothesis, emphasised hypoxia, hypovascularity, and hypocellularity, these do not fully account for the current understanding of the complex pathogenesis of ORNJ.

Q22. **Osteoradionecrosis management**

Answer: B. Curettage and removal of sequestrum is of benefit for early ORN of the jaw

Explanation: Conservative treatments, such as curettage and removal of sequestrum, are often employed in the early stages of ORNJ to manage symptoms and prevent progression. However, these methods are typically insufficient for advanced disease, which may require surgical interventions such as resection and reconstruction.

The PENTO regimen, combining pentoxifylline and tocopherol, improves vascular function and tissue oxygenation, addressing RIF, but does not directly promote osteoblast activity or bone regeneration (25).

Hyperbaric oxygen therapy has been debated for ORNJ management, with mixed evidence, and is not universally recommended. Surgical resection is reserved for refractory or severe cases, not as first-line therapy. Pharmacological approaches like the PENTO regimen are not limited to cases with pathological fractures and can be used in earlier stages.

Q23. **Management of impacted third molars**

Answer: D. Persistent apical infection is a potential complication that may necessitate reoperation after coronectomy.

Explanation: Coronectomy is a surgical technique that removes the crown of the mandibular third molar below the cementoenamel junction to preserve the roots and minimise the risk of IDN injury. Root migration is a well-documented phenomenon, occurring in 2% to 85.3% of cases, and while its consequences are often benign, reoperation may be required in cases of root exposure, persistent pain, or apical infection.

The procedure is indicated for mandibular third molars with a vital pulp and high risk of IDN injury. It is contraindicated in cases of non-vital pulp, caries extending into the pulp, mobile teeth, or associated tumours. CBCT is recommended for preoperative assessment in high-risk cases to confirm suitability for coronectomy (26).

Q24. **Antimicrobials for dentoalveolar infections**

Answer: C. Meropenem

Explanation: ESBL-producing organisms are resistant to most beta-lactam antibiotics, including penicillins, cephalosporins, and beta-lactam/beta-lactamase inhibitor combinations (e.g., amoxicillin-clavulanic acid or piperacillin-tazobactam). Carbapenems, such as meropenem, are the treatment of choice for serious infections caused by ESBL-producing bacteria due to their stability against ESBL-mediated hydrolysis and proven efficacy in severe infections. Vancomycin is not effective against gram-negative ESBL organisms but instead used in MRSA cases.

Q25. **Cavernous sinus thrombosis**

Answer: E. Mortality rate may be as high as 30%.

Explanation: Cavernous sinus thrombosis (CST) is a rare but life-threatening condition which can occur secondary to facial infections. The mortality rate for CST has decreased significantly since the introduction of antibiotics, but it can still be as high as 30%. Common causative organisms include Staphylococcus and Streptococcus species. MRI with venogram (MRV) is the preferred imaging method because it shows the absence of venous flow in the affected sinus. CST can be detected on CT but may be a subtle finding of increased density in the cavernous sinus. Treatment may involve a combination of antibiotics, surgical drainage and anticoagulation. Although dental infection may precipitate CST, infections involving the ethmoidal/sphenoidal sinuses and nasal furuncles are more commonly the cause.

Q26. **Peri-implant disease**

Answer: C. Peri-implant mucositis can be diagnosed based on the presence of inflammation without marginal bone loss.

Explanation: Peri-implant mucositis is a reversible inflammatory condition confined to the peri-implant mucosa, characterised by bleeding on gentle probing, redness, swelling, and occasionally suppuration, without evidence of marginal bone loss on radiographs. In this patient, the absence of bone loss and the presence of inflammation confirm the diagnosis of peri-implant mucositis. Peri-implantitis, in contrast, is associated with progressive bone loss, larger inflammatory lesions, and a higher density of osteoclast-activating cytokines such as IL1-alpha, TNF-alpha, and IL-6. In the absence of previous examination data (radiographs, probing measurements), a diagnosis of peri-implantitis can be made based on the combination of the presence of bleeding on probing depths ≥6 mm and a marginal bone level ≥3 mm apical to the most coronal portion of the endosseous part of the implant. The histological features of peri-implant mucositis include smaller inflammatory lesions compared to peri-implantitis and less involvement of B-cells and neutrophils (27).

Q27. **Apicectomy**

Answer: A. Apicectomy is indicated when there is a well-root-filled tooth with persistent periradicular disease and a high risk of root fracture from post removal.

Explanation: Apicectomy is indicated in cases where orthograde root canal treatment cannot be completed or has failed despite being carried out to guideline standards. For example, it is appropriate when periradicular disease persists in a well-root-filled tooth, particularly if root canal retreatment would risk structural integrity or involve destructive post removal. However, apicectomy is contraindicated if the coronal seal is poor, primary disease is not stabilised, or a combined periodontal-endodontic lesion is diagnosed. In addition, histopathological examination of periradicular tissues and cases with suspected root fractures or perforations are valid indications for the procedure. A poor coronal seal would compromise outcomes, even with a successful root-end resection.

Q28. **Apicectomy**

Answer: D. Root-end preparation should be performed using ultrasonic retrotips to facilitate proper sealing with a root-end filling material.

Explanation: When performing an apicectomy, careful attention to soft-tissue and osseous management, root-end resection, and filling materials is critical. Triangular, rectangular, or submarginal flaps are preferred for better access and healing; semilunar flaps are outdated due to scarring and poor visibility. Osteotomies should be kept small (less than 10 mm) to preserve success rates and promote faster healing. Root-end resection should be perpendicular and 3 mm deep to minimise exposed dentinal tubules, prevent leakage, and remove lateral canals and apical ramifications. Ultrasonic retrotips are superior to burs for root-end preparation, allowing deeper, parallel cuts and better visibility. MTA is the preferred root-end filling material due to its biocompatibility and bone regeneration properties, although zinc oxide eugenol-based materials such as IRM and super-EBA are also acceptable. Amalgam is no longer favoured due to inferior outcomes.

Q29. **Iatrogenic nerve injury**

Answer: D. Refer the patient to a specialist centre if there is no improvement in sensation by three months post-injury.

Explanation: Persistent numbness following lower third molar extraction is often due to injury to the inferior alveolar nerve. These injuries can be temporary or permanent, and proper management is crucial to ensure the best possible outcome. Early review and assessment of nerve function post-surgery are essential. If there is no evidence of recovery by three months, referral to a specialist centre is recommended to explore further treatment options, such as surgical decompression or repair. Failure to refer at this stage is considered a breach of duty and increases the risk of litigation. Immediate surgical intervention is not indicated unless imaging demonstrates canal disruption, and corticosteroids are not standard management in this context. It is essential to reassure patients but avoid dismissing their concerns, as this can lead to dissatisfaction and potential legal claims. Permanent nerve injuries may benefit from surgical repair, though the timing and success of these procedures can vary (28).

Q30. **Perioperative management for dentoalveolar surgery**

Answer: C. Aspirin irreversibly inhibits thromboxane A2.

Explanation: Aspirin works by inhibiting cyclooxygenase (COX), which is involved in the production of thromboxane A2, a substance critical for platelet aggregation and vasoconstriction. This inhibition is irreversible and lasts for the lifetime of the platelet, which is typically 3–7 days. Option A is incorrect because warfarin inhibits the activity of vitamin K-dependent clotting factors (II, VII, IX, and X), rather than increasing their activity. Option B is false because tranexamic acid inhibits, not promotes, fibrinolysis by preventing the conversion of plasminogen to plasmin. Option D is incorrect, as haemophilia A and B are characterised by a deficiency in clotting factors VIII and IX, respectively, leading to an increased risk of bleeding. Option E is false because clopidogrel irreversibly inhibits platelet aggregation by blocking the P2Y12 ADP receptor, and its use during surgery involving bleeding risk requires careful management depending on the bleeding risk.

Q31. **Coronectomy**

Answer: C. Root migration after coronectomy may occur, but it is not always clinically significant.

Explanation: Coronectomy is performed to minimise the risk of IDN injury by removing the crown while leaving the roots in place. Root migration is a known phenomenon, reported in 2% to 85.3% of cases. While it often does not result in complications, reoperation may be required in cases of root exposure, pain, or infection. The procedure is contraindicated in teeth with non-vital pulp, extensive caries, or pathology. Success rates range widely but are generally favourable, and ongoing monitoring is essential to ensure optimal outcomes.

Q32. ***Actinomyces israelii***

Answer: E. IV co-amoxiclav for four weeks followed by six months of amoxicillin

Explanation: "Sulphur granules" visible in the pus, which are characteristic of Actinomyces infection. Cervicofacial actinomycosis, most commonly caused by *Actinomyces israelii* (a gram-positive anaerobic bacteria), requires a prolonged course of antibiotic therapy. The recommended treatment is high-dose intravenous penicillin for 2–6 weeks, followed by oral penicillin or amoxicillin for 6–12 months. Surgical drainage may be necessary in cases of extensive abscess formation or persistent sinus tracts. Short-course antibiotics are insufficient due to the chronic, indolent nature of the infection. Surgical excision alone does not address the underlying infection.

11 Statistics and Research

QUESTIONS

Q1. A 60-year-old patient undergoes an MRI of the neck to evaluate for nodal metastasis in head and neck cancer. The MRI shows one lymph node that fits the radiological criteria for metastatic disease. Which of the following statements is correct regarding sensitivity, specificity, and predictive values in this context?

A. A highly sensitive test will have a low number of false positives.
B. A highly specific test will have a low number of false negatives.
C. Sensitivity is calculated as the number of true positives divided by the total number of people who have the disease.
D. Specificity is calculated as the number of true positives divided by the total number of people without the disease.
E. Positive predictive value (PPV) represents the proportion of positive test results that correctly identify disease.

Q2. A researcher is conducting a study comparing the outcomes of two surgical techniques for oral cavity cancer. They notice that one study group has a significantly higher number of participants lost to follow-up compared to the other group. What type of bias is most likely to be affecting this study?

A. Selection bias
B. Attrition bias
C. Measurement bias
D. Observer bias
E. Procedure bias

Q3. Which of the following statements regarding nonparametric statistical analysis is TRUE?

A. Nonparametric methods are highly influenced by outliers in the data.
B. Nonparametric methods can provide more detailed information than parametric methods.
C. Nonparametric methods are well-suited for small sample sizes.
D. Nonparametric methods are easier to compute, regardless of sample size.
E. Nonparametric methods rely heavily on assumptions about the population distribution.

Q4. A researcher is analysing the difference between two independent groups but discovers that the data is skewed and does not follow a normal distribution. Which of the following statistical tests is the most appropriate to use in this situation?

A. Two-sample t-test
B. Mann-Whitney U test
C. One-way ANOVA

DOI: 10.1201/9781003609308-12

D. Pearson correlation coefficient
E. Paired t-test

Q5. A researcher is studying the impact of a new surgical technique on the survival rate of patients with oral squamous cell carcinoma (OSCC) using a cohort study. The hazard ratio (HR) for recurrence of cancer is calculated. Which of the following is correct?
A. A hazard ratio (HR) of 1 indicates a higher risk of recurrence in the exposed group.
B. A hazard ratio (HR) of 0.5 means the exposed group has half the risk of recurrence, accounting for timing.
C. The hazard ratio (HR) can be used in both cohort and case-control studies.
D. A hazard ratio (HR) of 0.5 means the exposed group has twice the risk of recurrence, accounting for timing.
E. The hazard ratio (HR) cannot be used in survival studies.

Q6. You wish to conduct a study to investigate the relationship between smoking and the development of oral squamous cell carcinoma (OSCC). You decide to collect data on patients who have already been diagnosed with OSCC and compare their smoking history with a group of individuals who do not have OSCC. Which of the following study designs is being described?
A. Cross-sectional study
B. Case-control study
C. Prospective cohort study
D. Retrospective cohort study
E. Randomised controlled trial

Q7. An oral and maxillofacial surgeon is conducting a randomised controlled trial (RCT) to compare the effectiveness of two different surgical techniques for correcting mandibular fractures. Which of the following statements about randomised controlled trials is correct?
A. In an RCT, the results should be interpreted as showing a causal relationship only if the study is blinded.
B. Blinding is unnecessary in an RCT because randomisation alone eliminates bias.
C. In an RCT, outcome measures should be collected before randomisation to avoid bias in data interpretation.
D. The control group in an RCT receives no intervention so that there is a comparison for the intervention group.
E. Randomisation ensures that participants in the intervention and control groups have equal chances of being assigned to either group, reducing selection bias.

Q8. An oral and maxillofacial surgeon is evaluating the effectiveness of a new surgical technique for reducing postoperative complications in patients undergoing mandibular fracture surgery. In a clinical trial, the control event rate (CER) for complications in patients undergoing the standard procedure is 25%, and the experimental event rate (EER) for the new surgical technique is 15%. What is the number needed to treat (NNT) to prevent one additional postoperative complication using the new technique?

A. 5
B. 10
C. 8
D. 12
E. 15

ANSWERS AND EXPLANATIONS

Q1. **Sensitivity and specificity**

Explanation: Sensitivity is a measure of how good a test is at identifying those who actually have the disease. For example, if an MRI of the neck has a sensitivity of 75%, this means it misses some micrometastases (i.e., has a high number of false negatives). Conversely, specificity is a measure of how good a test is at identifying those who do not have the disease. If an MRI has a specificity of 95%, this means a positive finding on MRI is highly likely to represent true metastatic disease (29).

- **Correct answer (E)**: PPV is defined as the proportion of patients with a positive test result who are correctly diagnosed with the disease (PPV = true positives/[true positives + false positives]).
- **Option A**: A highly sensitive test has a low number of false negatives, not false positives.
- **Option B**: A highly specific test has a low number of false positives, not false negatives.
- **Option C**: While sensitivity does measure the ability to detect disease, it is calculated as true positives/(true positives + false negatives), representing only individuals who actually have the disease.
- **Option D**: Specificity is calculated as true negatives/(true negatives + false positives), and it applies to individuals without the disease.

Q2. **Types of bias**

Answer: B. Attrition bias

Explanation: Different types of biases exist that can affect study outcomes:

- **Attrition bias**: Arises from systematic differences in the number or characteristics of participants lost to follow-up between study groups. This difference can skew results, as the observed effect might be due to this imbalance rather than the intervention itself. In this scenario, the unequal loss to follow-up between the groups is a hallmark of attrition bias.
- **Selection bias**: An error in the process of selecting participants for the study and assigning them to particular arms of the study. It occurs with non-random sampling or treatment allocation of subjects such that the study population is not representative of the target population. Common strategies used to combat selection bias include appropriate randomisation of participants and ensuring the appropriate choice of comparison/reference group.
- **Measurement bias**: Involves inaccuracies in how data is collected or recorded, e.g. an inaccurate measurement tool. It occurs when information collected for use as a study variable is inaccurate. Measurement bias is effectively reduced when investigators use objective, standardised, and previously tested methods of data collection. The use of a placebo group can also be used to further decrease the chance of measurement bias.

- **Observer bias**: Occurs when assessors record outcomes differently, influenced by subjective judgement. Inter-rater reliability is the degree of agreement among independent observers who rate, code, or assess the same phenomenon. i.e. high inter-rater reliability ensures observer bias will not negatively impact results.
- **Procedure bias**: Occurs when subjects that have been allocated to different groups are not treated the same (apart from the variable being studied). Blinding of participants/investigators and the use of placebo are both viable strategies that can effectively reduce the chance of procedure bias.

Q3. **Nonparametric data interpretation**

Answer: C. Nonparametric methods are well-suited for small sample sizes.

Explanation: Statistical analysis is crucial for validating conclusions in medical research, transforming raw data into meaningful insights. While advancements in statistical software have made analyses more accessible, misuse or reliance on automated tools without understanding basic statistical concepts can lead to errors and undermine an article's credibility (30).

Understanding the normal distribution is essential for distinguishing between parametric and nonparametric data. In a normal distribution, the mean, mode, and median are equal and aligned at the peak of the curve. Additionally, 68% of the data falls within one standard deviation of the mean. This type of distribution can be fully described by just two parameters: the mean and standard deviation. Parametric data assumes this normal distribution, enabling the use of statistical methods based on these parameters. In contrast, nonparametric data does not rely on such assumptions and is used when data does not follow a normal distribution.

Nonparametric methods are particularly advantageous for small sample sizes, as they do not rely on assumptions about the population distribution and are less sensitive to outliers.

Nonparametric methods compute statistics based on signs or ranks, making them less influenced by outliers compared to parametric methods. Nonparametric methods provide limited information compared to parametric methods, as they do not allow for detailed population distribution analysis. While nonparametric methods are intuitive for small samples, computations can become complex for larger sample sizes. One of the main advantages of nonparametric methods is that they do not rely on assumptions about the population distribution.

Q4. **Statistical tests**

Answer: B. Mann-Whitney U test

Explanation: The Mann-Whitney U test is a nonparametric statistical test used to compare differences between two independent groups when the data does not meet the assumptions of normality. It evaluates differences in ranks rather than means, making it suitable for skewed or non-normal data.

- A. Two-sample t-test: Requires normally distributed data and assumes equal variance between groups.
- C. One-way ANOVA: Used for comparing means across more than two groups, assuming normality.
- D. Pearson correlation coefficient: Measures the linear relationship between two continuous variables, not group differences.
- E. Paired t-test: Used for paired or dependent data, not for comparing independent groups.

Summary of different tests for different purposes:

- **Assessing the difference between two groups**:
  - Parametric test: Two-sample t-test, assuming normal distribution and equal variance in the groups.
  - Nonparametric tests: Wilcoxon rank sum test, Mann-Whitney U test, and Kendall's S-test, used when the data does not meet parametric assumptions.
- **Assessing the difference between more than two groups**:
  - Parametric test: One-way ANOVA, which evaluates mean differences among groups assuming normality.
  - Nonparametric test: Kruskal-Wallis test, which compares ranks and is robust to non-normal distributions.
- **Measuring the strength of an association between two variables**:
  - Parametric method: Correlation coefficient (e.g., Pearson's), which assumes a linear relationship.
  - Nonparametric methods: Kendall's tau rank correlation and Spearman's rank correlation, which assess monotonic relationships without relying on normality.
- **Assessing the difference between paired observations**:
  - Parametric test: Paired t-test, assuming normal differences between paired data.
  - Nonparametric tests: Wilcoxon signed-rank test and Sign test, which are less sensitive to outliers and used when assumptions of the paired t-test are violated.

Q5. **Odds, risk, and hazard ratios**

Answer: B. A hazard ratio (HR) of 0.5 means the exposed group has half the risk of recurrence, accounting for timing.

Explanation:

- **Risk Ratio (RR)**:
  - Represents the simple ratio of the risk of an event occurring in the exposed group divided by the risk in the unexposed group.
  - Easy to interpret as a direct "times" comparison (e.g., a RR of 2 means the exposed group has twice the risk).
  - Can only be calculated directly from cohort studies where the exposure is assigned before the outcome is observed.
- **Odds Ratio (OR)**:
  - Represents the ratio of the odds of an event occurring in the exposed group divided by the odds in the unexposed group.
  - Often used in case-control studies where you can't directly calculate the RR.
  - Can overestimate the actual risk difference when the disease is not rare.
- **Hazard Ratio (HR)**:
  - Measures the instantaneous risk of an event occurring at any given time point during a study, taking into account the timing of events.
  - Primarily used in survival analysis where the outcome is time to a specific event (e.g., time to death).
  - Can be interpreted similarly to an RR but is more accurate when the event rate varies over time.

Interpreting the values:

- **Value of 1**: Indicates no difference in risk between groups.
- **Value greater than 1**: Indicates an increased risk in the exposed group.
- **Value less than 1**: Indicates a decreased risk in the exposed group.

What is the difference between risk and odds?

"Risk" refers to the probability of occurrence of an event or outcome. Statistically, risk = chance of the outcome of interest/all possible outcomes. The term "odds" is often used instead of risk. "Odds" refers to the probability of occurrence of an event/probability of the event not occurring.

Q6. **Study design**

Answer: B. Case-control study

Explanation:

- **Case-control study** compares individuals with the disease (cases) to those without the disease (controls) to identify risk factors (e.g., smoking). This design is typically retrospective, as it looks back at past exposures to determine associations.
- **Cross-sectional study** provides a snapshot of the population at a single point in time and is used to measure the prevalence of disease, not risk factors or exposures.
- **Prospective cohort study** follows individuals over time to track the development of a disease based on exposures.
- **Retrospective cohort study** looks back at past exposures in individuals who already have or do not have the outcome of interest.
- **RCT** involves assigning participants to different groups to test the effects of an intervention, not used for studying risk factors like smoking.

Q7. **Randomised controlled trial (RCT)**

Answer: E. Randomisation ensures that participants in the intervention and control groups have equal chances of being assigned to either group, reducing selection bias.

Explanation: Randomisation minimises selection bias by ensuring that each participant has an equal chance of being assigned to either the treatment or control group, which increases the reliability of the results. The presence or absence of blinding does not invalidate the ability to draw causal conclusions in an RCT. Blinding helps prevent performance bias and detection bias, ensuring that the treatment or outcome assessment is not influenced by knowledge of group assignment. In an RCT, outcome measures are collected after randomisation to assess the effects of the intervention and avoid introduction of bias. In an RCT, the control group often receives a placebo or standard treatment, not necessarily no intervention, to provide a valid comparison for the new treatment.

Q8. **Number needed to treat**

Answer: B. 10

Explanation: The NNT is the number of patients you need to treat to prevent one additional negative outcome (death, stroke, etc.). For example, if a drug has a NNT of 5, it means you have to treat five people with the drug to prevent one additional complication/bad outcome (31).

To calculate the NNT, we first need to determine the Absolute Risk Reduction (ARR):

$$\text{ARR} = \text{CER} - \text{EER} = 0.25 - 0.15 = 0.10\left(10\%\right).$$

Then, we calculate the NNT:

$$\text{NNT} = 1/\text{ARR} = 1/0.10 = 10.$$

The correct answer is **10** (NNTs are always rounded up to the nearest whole number).

References

1. Maghami, E, Ismaila, N, Alvarez, A, Chernock, R, Duvvuri, U, Geiger, J, et al. Diagnosis and Management of Squamous Cell Carcinoma of Unknown Primary in the Head and Neck: ASCO Guideline. *JCO*. 2020 August; 38(22):2570–96.
2. Zanoni, DK, Patel, SG, Shah, JP. Changes in the 8th Edition of the American Joint Committee on Cancer (AJCC) Staging of Head and Neck Cancer: Rationale and Implications. *Curr Oncol Rep*. 2019 April 17;21(6):52.
3. NG36: Recommendations | Cancer of the upper aerodigestive tract: assessment and management in people aged 16 and over | Guidance | NICE [Internet]. NICE; 2016 [cited 2025 February 17]. Available from: https://www.nice.org.uk/guidance/ng36/chapter/Recommendations#treatment-of-early-stage-disease
4. D'Cruz, AK, Vaish, R, Kapre, N, Dandekar, M, Gupta, S, Hawaldar, R, et al. Elective versus Therapeutic Neck Dissection in Node-Negative Oral Cancer. *N Engl J Med*. 2015 August 6;373(6):521–9.
5. Arganbright, JM, Tsue, TT, Girod, DA, Militsakh, ON, Sykes, KJ, Markey, J, et al. Outcomes of the Osteocutaneous Radial Forearm Free Flap for Mandibular Reconstruction. *JAMA Otolaryngol Head Neck Surg*. 2013 February;139(2):168–72.
6. Jiang, X, Li, Y, Chen, N, Zhou, M, He, L. Corticosteroids for Preventing Postherpetic Neuralgia. *Cochrane Database Syst. Rev*. 2023;12(12):CD005582. DOI: 10.1002/14651858.CD005582.pub5/full
7. Brown, S, Jones, G, Rawnsley, S. Observing Teaching. SEDA Paper 79 [Internet]. SEDA Administrator, Gala House, 3 Raglan Rd; 1993 [cited 2020 May 1]. Available from: https://eric.ed.gov/?id=ED376756
8. Long, JA. A Method of Monocanalicular Silicone Intubation. *Ophthalmic Surg*. 1988 March;19(3):204–5.
9. Bottini, GB, Roccia, F, Sobrero, F. Management of Pediatric Mandibular Condyle Fractures: A Literature Review. *J Clin Med*. 2024 January;13(22):6921.
10. Ducruet, AF, Albuquerque, FC, Crowley, RW, McDougall, CG. The Evolution of Endovascular Treatment of Carotid Cavernous Fistulas: A Single-Center Experience. *World Neurosurg*. 2013 November;80(5):538–48.
11. Evans, BT, Webb, AAC. Post-Traumatic Orbital Reconstruction: Anatomical Landmarks and the Concept of the Deep Orbit. *Br J Oral Maxillofac Surg*. 2007 April;45(3):183–9.
12. Koch, M, Iro, H. Salivary Duct Stenosis: Diagnosis and Treatment. *Acta Otorhinolaryngol Ital*. 2017 April;37(2):132–41.
13. Koch, M, Mantsopoulos, K, Müller, S, Sievert, M, Iro, H. Treatment of Sialolithiasis: What Has Changed? An Update of the Treatment Algorithms and a Review of the Literature. *J Clin Med*. 2021 December 31;11(1):231.
14. Lazaridou, M, Iliopoulos, C, Antoniades, K, Tilaveridis, I, Dimitrakopoulos, I, Lazaridis, N. Salivary Gland Trauma: A Review of Diagnosis and Treatment. *Craniomaxillofac Trauma Reconstr*. 2012 December;5(4):189–96.
15. Obwegeser, HL, Makek, MS. Hemimandibular hyperplasia—hemimandibular elongation. *J Maxillofac Surg*. 1986 August;14(4):183–208.
16. Martelli-Junior, H, Chaves, MR, Swerts, MSO, de Miranda, RT, Bonan, PRF, Coletta, RD. Clinical and Genetic Features of Van der Woude Syndrome in Two Large Families in Brazil. *Cleft Palate Craniofac J*. 2007 May;44(3):239–43.

17. Shprintzen, RJ. The Implications of the Diagnosis of Robin Sequence. *Cleft Palate Craniofac J*. 1992 May;29(3):205–9.
18. Tse, R. Unilateral Cleft Lip: Principles and Practice of Surgical Management. *Semin Plast Surg*. 2012 November;26(4):145–55.
19. Stal, S, Brown, RH, Higuera, S, Hollier, LH, Byrd, HS, Cutting, CB, et al. Fifty Years of the Millard Rotation-Advancement: Looking Back and Moving Forward. *Plast Reconstr Surg*. 2009 April;123(4):1364–77.
20. McCain, JP, Sanders, B, Koslin, MG, Quinn, JH, Peters, PB, Indresano, AT. Temporomandibular Joint Arthroscopy: A 6-Year Multicenter Retrospective Study of 4,831 Joints. *J Oral Maxillofac Surg*. 1992 September;50(9):926–30.
21. Paolantonio, EG, Ludovici, N, Saccomanno, S, La Torre, G, Grippaudo, C. Association Between Oral Habits, Mouth Breathing and Malocclusion in Italian Preschoolers. *Eur J Paediatr Dent*. 2019 September;20(3):204–8.
22. Sharma, S, Vashistha, A, Chugh, A, Kumar, D, Bihani, U, Trehan, M, et al. Pediatric Mandibular Fractures: A Review. *Int J Clin Pediatr Dent*. 2009;2(2):1–5.
23. Wolford, LM, Morales-Ryan, CA, García-Morales, P, Perez, D. Surgical Management of Mandibular Condylar Hyperplasia Type 1. *Proc (Bayl Univ Med Cent)*. 2009 October;22 (4):321–9.
24. Scenario: Apixaban | Management | Anticoagulation - oral | CKS | NICE [Internet]. [cited 2025 February 17]. Available from: https://cks.nice.org.uk/topics /anticoagulation-oral/management/apixaban/
25. Arqueros-Lemus, M, Mariño-Recabarren, D, Niklander, S, Martínez-Flores, R, Moraga, V. Pentoxifylline and Tocopherol for the Treatment of Osteoradionecrosis of the Jaws. A Systematic Review. *Med Oral Patol Oral Cir Bucal*. 2023 May;28(3):e293–300.
26. Martin, A, Perinetti, G, Costantinides, F, Maglione, M. Coronectomy as a Surgical Approach to Impacted Mandibular Third Molars: A Systematic Review. *Head Face Med*. 2015 May;10;11:9.
27. Heitz-Mayfield, LJA. Peri-Implant Mucositis and Peri-Implantitis: Key Features and Differences. *Br Dent J*. 2024 May;236(10):791–4.
28. Smith, KG. Repair of Nerves Injured During Dental and Oral Surgery Procedures. *FDJ*. 2011 October;2(4):158–63.
29. Monaghan, TF, Rahman, SN, Agudelo, CW, Wein, AJ, Lazar, JM, Everaert, K, et al. Foundational Statistical Principles in Medical Research: Sensitivity, Specificity, Positive Predictive Value, and Negative Predictive Value. *Medicina (Kaunas)*. 2021 May 16;57(5):503.
30. Nahm, FS. Nonparametric Statistical Tests for the Continuous Data: The Basic Concept and the Practical Use. *Korean J Anesthesiol*. 2016 February;69(1):8–14.
31. Sackett, DL, Straus, SE, Scott Richardson, W, William Rosenberg, R Haynes, B. *Evidence-Based Medicine: How to Practice and Teach EBM*. 2nd ed. Churchill Livingstone; 2000.

Index